Complications in Orthopaedics
Total Hip Arthroplasty

Edited by
Craig J. Della Valle, MD
Associate Professor
Department of Orthopaedic Surgery
Rush University Medical Center
Chicago, Illinois

Series Editor
Peter C. Amadio, MD
Mayo Clinic
Rochester, Minnesota

Published by the
American Academy of Orthopaedic Surgeons
6300 North River Road
Rosemont, IL 60018

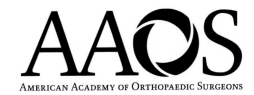

AMERICAN ACADEMY OF ORTHOPAEDIC SURGEONS

First Edition
Copyright © 2009 by the
American Academy of Orthopaedic Surgeons

ISBN   10: 0-89203-500-5
ISBN   13: 978-0-89203-500-7

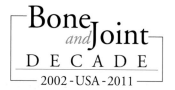

Contributors

Kevin J. Bozic, MD, MBA
Associate Professor in Residence
Department of Orthopaedic Surgery and
    Institute for Policy and Practice
University of California, San Francisco
San Francisco, California

Joshua J. Jacobs, MD
Professor and Chairman
Department of Orthopaedic Surgery
Rush University Medical Center
Chicago, Illinois

Brian A. Klatt, MD
Assistant Professor, Joint Reconstruction
Department of Orthopaedic Surgery
University of Pittsburgh Physicians
University of Pittsburgh
Pittsburgh, Pennsylvania

Gregg R. Klein, MD
Attending Physician
Hartzband Joint Replacement Institute
Hackensack University Medical Center
Hackensack, New Jersey

Brett Levine, MD, MS
Attending Physician
Midwest Orthopaedic Center
Peoria, Illinois

David Manning, MD
Assistant Professor
Department of Orthopaedics and Adult
    Reconstruction
University of Chicago Medical Center
University of Chicago
Chicago, Illinois

Javad Parvizi, MD
Professor
Department of Orthopaedic Surgery
Rothman Institute at Thomas Jefferson
    University
Philadelphia, Pennsylvania

Michael D. Ries, MD
Professor of Orthopaedic Surgery
University of California, San Francisco
San Francisco, California

Todd Sekundiak, MD, FRCSC
Assistant Professor
Department of Orthopaedic Surgery
Creighton University
Omaha, Nebraska

Scott M. Sporer, MD, MS
Assistant Professor of Orthopaedic Surgery
Rush University Medical Center
Chicago, Illinois

Thomas Parker Vail, MD
Professor and Chairman
Department of Orthopaedic Surgery
University of California, San Francisco
San Francisco, California

Contents

Preface

Despite the overwhelming overall success of total hip arthroplasty, it is inevitable that perioperative complications will sometimes occur. As physicians, we are taught to do no harm, and thus managing such problems is one of the most challenging parts of our jobs. It is said that physicians are paid not for the cases that go well—because the inherent satisfaction of substantially improving a patient's quality of life is payment enough—but for the patients who do poorly.

A thorough understanding of the most commonly encountered complications associated with total hip arthroplasty is paramount to their prevention. Similarly, a thorough knowledge of appropriate treatment options is critical to minimizing morbidity when complications do occur. The goals of this monograph, therefore, are threefold: to help the practicing orthopaedic surgeon recognize the most common perioperative problems encountered following total hip arthroplasty, to provide strategies for preventing such problems, and to present treatment algorithms for the management of complications that occur despite the surgeon's best efforts.

I would like to extend my thanks to the team of authors who shared their expertise and time to help create this monograph. I also would like to thank the staff of the Publications Department at the American Academy of Orthopaedic Surgeons, whose efforts made this publication a reality.

Craig J. Della Valle, MD
Editor

Chapter 1

PERIPHERAL NERVE INJURY

Scott M. Sporer, MD

CASE PRESENTATION

History

A 44-year-old woman presented with increasing pain and discomfort in both hips. She began experiencing hip pain as a child and was diagnosed at that time with bilateral hip dysplasia. The patient had been relatively active up until the last several years, but at the time of presentation she required the use of a cane for daily activities. She had tried nonsteroidal anti-inflammatory drugs in the past with no benefit.

On physical examination, the patient ambulated with the assistance of a cane. A Trendelenburg gait pattern was noted, as well as an antalgic component on the right side. Hip range of motion was 95° of flexion, full extension, internal rotation to 20°, and external rotation to 40° on the right side; the range of motion on the left side was similar. She had pain at the extremes of motion. A passive straight-leg raise test elicited no pain. Motor testing demonstrated hip flexor strength grade 3/5 and hip abductor strength grade 4/5. Radiographs, including an AP pelvic view and AP and lateral views of the right hip, demonstrated Crowe type IV bilateral hip dysplasia (**Figure 1**).

Initial Management

The patient was counseled on surgical and nonsurgical management options, and she elected to proceed with surgical intervention. A staged bilateral total hip arthroplasty (THA) was planned with an interval of 4 weeks between hips.

A THA of the right hip was performed via a posterior approach. The acetabular component was placed in the anatomic hip center. Severe hip dysplasia was present, so a subtrochanteric shortening osteotomy approximately 6 cm in length was performed to minimize risk of neurologic injury (**Figure 2**).

---

*Scott M. Sporer, MD, or the department with which he is affiliated has received research or institutional support, miscellaneous nonincome support, commercially derived honoraria, or other nonresearch-related funding from Zimmer and is a consultant for or an employee of Zimmer.

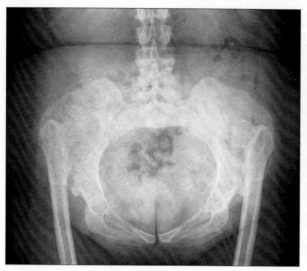

Figure 1 Preoperative radiograph demonstrating Crowe type IV dysplasia. Note the complete dislocation of the femoral heads bilaterally with proximal migration.

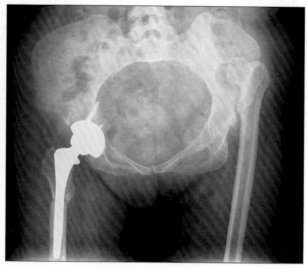

Figure 2 Postoperative radiograph demonstrating cementless femoral and acetabular components. Note the subtrochanteric osteotomy used to minimize risk of neurologic injury.

The patient tolerated the procedure well, and the neurovascular examination conducted in the recovery room was normal.

On postoperative day 2, an acute loss of motor and sensory function developed in the patient's right foot. This occurred when she was out of bed and sitting in a chair with her knee straight. She was brought back to bed immediately and positioned with the head of the bed level and her right knee flexed. Motor and sensory function improved within 15 minutes, but the symptoms recurred approximately 8 hours later when she attempted to sit up in bed for breakfast. At this time, the thigh on the affected side was soft and the patient's hemoglobin remained stable. She was again placed in a position to minimize the tension on the sciatic nerve, and the symptoms improved. She continued to describe painful dysesthesia, for which she was started on gabapentin.

Outcome

The patient's symptoms of dysesthesia improved over the subsequent 4 weeks. At approximately 2 years' follow-up, the patient reported no residual neurologic effects.

DISCUSSION
Recognizing the Problem and High-Risk Situations

Neurologic injury following elective THA is a devastating complication for both the patient and surgeon and remains a substantial cause of orthopaedic-related litigation. Although there is no way to completely eliminate this complication, joint arthroplasty surgeons should be aware of preoperative characteristics and situations that place a patient at an elevated risk.

A neurologic injury can be classified as an injury either to a peripheral nerve or to the central nervous system. Peripheral nerve injuries can occur either near the surgical site or at a distant location, such as the contralateral limb or the upper extremity. This discussion will focus on peripheral nerve injuries near the surgical site because this represents the most common and most vexing problem seen by joint arthroplasty surgeons.

The prevalence of peripheral nerve injuries following all hip arthroplasty procedures is approximately 1%.[1] Subclinical injuries, however, may occur in as many as 70% of patients undergoing THA.[2]

Injury to the sciatic nerve accounts for 90% of peripheral nerve injuries, followed by the femoral, superior gluteal, and obturator nerve. The peroneal division of the sciatic nerve is the most commonly injured portion of the sciatic nerve. Schmalzried and associates[3] reported that more than 94% of sciatic nerve injuries involved the peroneal portion of the sciatic nerve, whereas isolated tibial nerve injuries were rare. One hypothesis for the higher risk of damage to the peroneal portion of the sciatic nerve is that at the level of the hip, the fascicles of the peroneal division are denser, making it more susceptible to injury. Other factors, such as the closer proximity to retractors compared to the tibial division, the relative tethering of the nerve between the sciatic notch and the fibular head, and the compression of the nerve between the ischial tuberosity and femoral insertion of the gluteus maximus, may contribute to the higher risk of injury.[4,5] Preoperative risk factors for damage to the sciatic nerve include female sex, hip dysplasia, revision surgery, combined nerve root compression of the lumbar spine, or peripheral neuropathy.[3,6] Other series suggest that a posterior surgical approach, deficient posterior wall, excision of heterotopic bone, lengthening of the extremity, and the use of cementless femoral implants may result in a higher risk of sciatic injury.[7]

Femoral nerve injuries are much less common following THA; in one large series, they accounted for 13% of peripheral nerve injuries.[1] Anatomically, the femoral nerve is located deep to the rectus femoris and remains lateral to the femoral artery and vein at the level of the hip. Direct compression of the nerve is the most common etiology and can easily occur if a retractor is placed anterior to the rectus. An anterior surgical approach, deficient anterior acetabular bone, and a previously released or absent psoas tendon have been shown to be risk factors for this injury.

Superior gluteal nerve injuries are becoming more common as more surgeons elect to use a gluteal-splitting approach for routine primary THA.[8] The superior gluteal nerve innervates the gluteus medius, gluteus minimus, and the tensor fascia lata. This nerve is at risk when the extension into the gluteus medius extends more than 5 cm beyond the tip of the greater trochanter. Although injury to the sciatic nerve is the most common nerve injury reported following THA, it is likely that superior gluteal injuries are actually much more common. Ramesh and associates[8] demonstrated a 23% prevalence of injury following THA using a Hardinge approach. The difficulty in identifying superior gluteal injuries postoperatively is that patients present with abductor weakness and a Trendelenburg gait pattern similar to patients with an abductor avulsion.

Treatment

The successful treatment of any neurologic injury relies on a prompt clinical diagnosis. The surgeon must evaluate and document the neurologic status of the patient preoperatively, including an evaluation of the patient's mental status as well as sensory and motor function in both the upper and lower extremities. A repeat examination should be performed immediately in the recovery room, as soon as the patient is able to follow commands. If an immediate postoperative neurologic examination is not performed, it is difficult to differentiate a delayed nerve injury (such as is described in the case presentation) from an injury that occurred intraoperatively. The patient and family should also be counseled immediately if a nerve injury is identified so that they can help in the immediate postoperative monitoring of the extremity.

Physical examination to evaluate the sciatic nerve should include both the peroneal and tibial distributions. Motor function of the peroneal nerve can be assessed by placing the foot in a neutral dorsiflexion/plantar flexion position and asking the patient to raise the great toe and ankle; this will assess motor function of the extensor hallucis longus and tibialis anterior muscles. It is not sufficient to have patients move their toes with the foot in a plantar flexed position because rebound extension may be perceived as peroneal function. Sensory function of the peroneal nerve can be assessed by testing sensation in the first dorsal web space. Ideally, the patient should be able to discriminate light touch as well as sharp/dull. Motor function of the tibial nerve can be assessed by having the patient flex the great toe and plantar flex the foot against resistance; sensory function of the tibial nerve can be tested on the plantar surface of the foot.

The treatment of a postoperative sciatic nerve palsy depends on the etiology and the time at which the palsy was identified. Unfortunately, the etiology of most sciatic nerve palsies is unknown.[3] Ultimately, the surgeon must decide if acute surgical intervention will result in a greater chance of recovery. Once a sciatic nerve palsy is identified, all tight bandages, straps from an abduction pillow, or compression stockings should be removed. Patients who have received regional anesthesia (long-acting spinal or epidural) must be monitored closely because a palsy may go unrecognized if sensory and motor weakness is attributed to residual effects of the anesthesia. All patients should be placed in a position that will allow the hip to be extended and the knee flexed to minimize tension on the sciatic nerve. Postoperative radiographs can determine if the surgery resulted in substantial leg lengthening. Several authors have suggested that isolated modular femoral head exchange to shorten the extremity may result in neurologic improvement.[9,10] Postoperative radiographs should also be evaluated for component position and the location of any bone graft or supplemental screws. A CT scan or Judet radiographic views may be helpful if mechanical impingement is suspected. If a mechanical cause of injury is suspected, the patient should be brought back to the operating room as soon as medically feasible.

Late neurologic injury can occur from an expanding hematoma near the surgical site or near the epidural space. The circumference of the patient's thigh should be measured and compared with the contralateral extremity. Serial measurements may demonstrate clinical signs of an expanding hematoma. The patient's hemoglobin and level of anticoagulation should also be monitored to determine whether a sudden drop in hemoglobin or a sudden rise in the level of anticoagulation occurred. Imaging tools such as CT and ultrasound have been used to quantify the size of a hematoma.

If an epidural hematoma is suspected, an urgent MRI scan should be performed; this is the most sensitive study to detect an expanding epidural hematoma. Immediate neurosurgical consultation should be considered in patients with evolving neurologic symptoms, especially if multiple nerve roots appear to be affected. Delayed neurologic injury also can occur as a result of patient positioning, as described in the case presentation. Hip flexion and knee extension result in a relative lengthening of the sciatic nerve. Fleming and associates[11] evaluated the strain on the sciatic nerve in 10 patients undergoing primary THA. A mean 26% increase in strain was observed during flexion of the hip and extension of the knee. This degree of strain can exceed the threshold before neuralgic symptoms become clinically apparent, especially when surgery causes limb lengthening.

When no cause can be identified for a sciatic nerve palsy, the patient should be followed closely to ensure that the neurologic insult does not progress. Bracing of the foot with an ankle-foot orthosis (AFO) should be started in the early postoperative period. An AFO can assist with ambulation and minimize the chance of development of a plantar flexion contracture of the ipsilateral ankle. Patients who have a complete sciatic nerve palsy must be counseled on the importance of skin care to minimize the risk of ulceration. Electromyography and nerve conduction velocity studies should be considered in patients with residual motor or sensory defects at 4 to 6 weeks postoperatively. These studies are helpful in identifying the location of the injury and provide an assessment of a baseline level of function. Many patients with a sciatic nerve palsy report painful dysesthesias that can develop into a chronic regional pain syndrome, and patients often find these symptoms worse than residual motor weakness. Collaboration with a physician specializing in chronic pain should be considered early on, as the use of tricyclic antidepressants, gabapentin, or pregabalin can be considered to prevent the development of a chronic regional pain syndrome.

The treatment of a femoral nerve palsy, like a sciatic nerve palsy, depends on the etiology of the palsy. Observation is generally recommended because most femoral nerve palsies are caused by excessive retraction during the surgical approach. Other inciting causes, such as impingement from extruded cement, a bone screw, or an expanding hematoma, must be considered, however, and surgical intervention to relieve the source of impingement on the nerve should be considered. Femoral nerve palsies can result in profound quadriceps weakness, resulting in difficulty with ambulation. In these situations, a knee immobilizer or a long-leg drop-lock brace can be beneficial until motor strength improves.

The clinical outcome following a nerve injury depends on both the mechanism and the severity of the injury, as well as patient-related factors. The specific nerve injured, the degree of the injury, the zone of the injury, the distance from the injury to the end organ, and the environment surrounding the nerve all have been shown to be important prognostic indicators for recovery.[4] Patient-related factors include age, neurologic comorbidities (diabetes, lumbar spine disease, alcoholism), and medical comorbidities (smoking, steroid use). Farrell and associates[7] reported a rate of complete motor strength recovery of only 36% in patients who initially had complete loss of motor or sensation. They demonstrated a rate of complete motor strength recovery of only 39% in patients who initially had only a partial loss of strength. Schmalzried and associates[1] evaluated 228 nerve palsies and reported that 41% of patients were asymptomatic, 44% were left with mild residual deficits, and 15% had major deficits. The return of some motor function within the first 2 weeks postoperatively and the presence of some sensory function appear to be good prognostic indicators.[1] The outcome of femoral nerve palsies is controversial. Although many authors believe the prognosis for recovery is better with a femoral nerve injury compared to a sciatic nerve injury,[1] others have shown a very low prevalence of complete recovery.[12]

Prevention of Peripheral Nerve Injury Following THA

The risk of peripheral nerve injury following THA cannot be eliminated, but various preoperative, intraoperative, and postoperative factors should be considered to minimize the risk of this complication. Preoperatively, patients who have ipsilateral peripheral neuropathy, lumbar disk disease, or hip dysplasia, or who require lengthening of the limb are at a higher risk of injury. These patients should be counseled and additional care should be taken in the operating room to minimize any excessive tension on the nerve. Release of the gluteus maximus tendon is suggested in these patients because the femoral insertion of the gluteus maximus can act as a tether to the sciatic nerve.[5]

Surgeons must be familiar with the surrounding anatomy relevant to the chosen surgical approaches. A posterior approach places the sciatic nerve at

increased risk, whereas an anterior or lateral approach places the femoral and superior gluteal nerves, respectively, at an increased risk. All retractors should be placed either against bone or against soft tissue that is adjacent to the nerve. The sciatic nerve can be palpated during a posterior approach, but formal exploration is not recommended. The surgical limb should be maintained in a position that reduces the stress on the nerve most at risk; a position of hip extension and knee flexion is recommended when a posterior approach is chosen.

The role of somatosensory-evoked potentials (SSEPs) applied to the lower extremities and monitored intraoperatively (as is done in some spinal procedures) remains controversial. There is little clinical evidence to suggest that this method of monitoring nerve function will decrease the incidence of nerve injury. SSEPs are also cost and time intensive and remain impractical for routine total joint arthroplasty.

Acetabular screw fixation is commonly used to supplement initial component fixation. The quadrant system described by Wasielewski and associates[13] can identify a "safe zone" for screw placement (**Figure 3**). The posterior superior quadrant minimizes the chance of neurovascular compromise and is recommended for routine primary THA.

Limb lengthening undoubtedly places a nerve at an increased risk of injury. The limb may be lengthened either inadvertently during THA or intentionally in situations such as hip dysplasia, congenital leg-length inequality, or prior trauma. Patient comorbidities (diabetes, smoking history, associated peripheral neuropathy), the chronicity of the shortened extremity, and the amount of intraoperative lengthening are all important risk factors to consider when determining if the extremity can safely be lengthened. A patient with a history of a traumatic event that led to the leg-length inequality is not at the same level of risk for neurologic injury as the patient with a congenital short limb. In the former situation, the nerve was at one time the "appropriate" length, whereas in the latter case, the nerve was never the desired length and any lengthening of the limb can lead to damage. It has been suggested that a limb can be lengthened either 4 cm or 6% of its length, whichever is less, without causing a sensory/motor deficit. Other surgeons have found no statistical correlation between

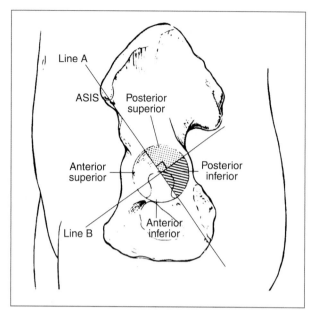

Figure 3 The safe quadrant as described by Wasielewski. ASIS = anterior superior iliac spine. (Reproduced with permission from Wasielewski RC, Cooperstein LA, Kruger MP, Rubash HE: Acetabular anatomy and the transacetabular fixation of screws in total hip arthroplasty. *J Bone Joint Surg Am* 1990;72:501-508.)

the amount of limb lengthening and the incidence of nerve damage.[14] A subtrochanteric osteotomy should be considered in patients with hip dysplasia if significant limb lengthening is anticipated. Alternatively, a trochanteric advancement may provide improved soft-tissue tension while decreasing the need for limb lengthening in patients requiring hip revision.

CASE SUMMARY
Management

The patient described in the initial case report was at a very high preoperative risk of nerve injury. She was counseled preoperatively about the complexity of the surgery and the multiple reasons why she was at a high risk of postoperative neurologic compromise. The patient had Crowe type IV hip dysplasia with severe shortening of her extremity. The preoperative plan was to place her acetabular component at the level of the true hip center, which would have resulted in lengthening her leg approximately 10 cm. A 6-cm corrective osteotomy was performed to allow the hip to be reduced yet minimize the tension on the sciatic nerve. The patient's neurologic status was evaluated preoperatively and immediately postoperatively. Despite a normal examination, sensory and motor loss developed on the second postoperative day.

A history of the events preceding the nerve palsy suggested that the relative lengthening of the sciatic nerve during positioning (hip flexed, knee extended) caused the neurologic compromise. Placing the patient immediately in a position that decreased the strain on the nerve resulted in improvement. The patient did describe painful dysesthesia for approximately 4 weeks postoperatively, during which time gabapentin was prescribed.

Outcome

At 2 years' follow-up, the patient remains asymptomatic, with full recovery of sensory and motor function.

STRATEGIES TO MINIMIZE COMMON COMPLICATIONS

Preoperative counseling is crucial in clinical scenarios that place a patient at an increased risk of neurologic injury. Preoperative knowledge of the potential for postoperative sensory or motor loss will not only help patients make an informed decision as to whether or not they wish to proceed with surgery but also prepare patients if an injury does occur. All preexisting medical comorbidities and neurologic injuries should be optimized before surgery, but the risk attributed to these conditions remains and is beyond the control of the orthopaedic surgeon. Actions that can be taken to minimize risk factors include appropriate preoperative templating to avoid inadvertent limb lengthening, making sure that femoral and acetabular retractors are placed against bone throughout the procedure, and maintaining the limb in a position that minimizes tension on the nerve at greatest risk given the surgical approach. Surgeons should also be aware of "safe" positions for the placement of acetabular screws and should avoid plunging during drilling of the bone. A thorough neurologic examination upon completion of the surgical procedure is crucial to promptly identify an intraoperative neurologic injury. Successful long-term recovery depends on prompt recognition and early intervention when a cause can be identified.

REFERENCES

1. Schmalzried TP, Noordin S, Amstutz HC: Update on nerve palsy associated with total hip replacement. *Clin Orthop Relat Res* 1997;344:188-206.

2. Weber ER, Daube JR, Coventry MB: Peripheral neuropathies associated with total hip arthroplasty. *J Bone Joint Surg Am* 1976;58:66-69.

3. Schmalzried TP, Amstutz HC, Dorey FJ: Nerve palsy associated with total hip replacement: Risk factors and prognosis. *J Bone Joint Surg Am* 1991;73:1074-1080.

4. DeHart MM, Riley LH Jr: Nerve injuries in total hip arthroplasty. *J Am Acad Orthop Surg* 1999;7:101-111.

5. Hurd JL, Potter HG, Dua V, Ranawat CS: Sciatic nerve palsy after primary total hip arthroplasty: A new perspective. *J Arthroplasty* 2006;21:796-802.

6. Johanson NA, Pellicci PM, Tsairis P, Salvati EA: Nerve injury in total hip arthroplasty. *Clin Orthop Relat Res* 1983;179:214-222.

7. Farrell CM, Springer BD, Haidukewych GJ, Morrey BF: Motor nerve palsy following primary total hip arthroplasty. *J Bone Joint Surg Am* 2005;87:2619-2625.

8. Ramesh M, O'Byrne JM, McCarthy N, Jarvis A, Mahalingham K, Cashman WF: Damage to the superior gluteal nerve after the Hardinge approach to the hip. *J Bone Joint Surg Br* 1996;78:903-906.

9. Pritchett JW: Nerve injury and limb lengthening after hip replacement: Treatment by shortening. *Clin Orthop Relat Res* 2004;418:168-171.

10. Silbey MB, Callaghan JJ: Sciatic nerve palsy after total hip arthroplasty: Treatment by modular neck shortening. *Orthopedics* 1991;14:351-352.

11. Fleming P, Lenehan B, O'Rourke S, McHugh P, Kaar K, McCabe JP: Strain on the human sciatic nerve in vivo during movement of the hip and knee. *J Bone Joint Surg Br* 2003;85:363-365.

12. Hudson AR, Hunter GA, Waddell JP: Iatrogenic femoral nerve injuries. *Can J Surg* 1979;22:62-66.

13. Wasielewski RC, Cooperstein LA, Kruger MP, Rubash HE: Acetabular anatomy and the transacetabular fixation of screws in total hip arthroplasty. *J Bone Joint Surg Am* 1990;72:501-508.

14. Eggli S, Hankemayer S, Muller ME: Nerve palsy after leg lengthening in total replacement arthroplasty for developmental dysplasia of the hip. *J Bone Joint Surg Br* 1999;81:843-845.

Chapter 2

VASCULAR INJURY

Gregg R. Klein, MD
*Craig J. Della Valle, MD

INTRODUCTION
Anatomic Considerations

Vascular injury has been documented at almost every part of a total hip arthroplasty (THA).[1] The reported incidence of vascular injury ranges from 0.1% to 0.2%.[2] The external iliac and common femoral vessels are the most commonly injured.[3]

The external iliac vessels run down the medial border of the psoas muscle, with the muscle interposed between the anterior column of the acetabulum and the vessels. Injury to the external iliac vessels has been described from patient positioning through implant insertion. External iliac injury is often a direct result of retractor placement over the anterior column of the acetabulum. Retractors positioned too medially, especially distally, may cause direct penetration of the vessel or a stretching or tearing of the vessels.[1] It has been hypothesized that more proximal placement may be safer because there is more muscle proximally than distally. Reaming through the medial wall of the acetabulum also may injure the iliac vessels.[2,3] Although less common today, cement extrusion into the pelvis may result in thermal injury to the vessels. Finally, screw placement in the anterior superior quadrant places the iliac artery at risk.

The common femoral vessels lie anterior and medial to the hip capsule. They are direct extensions of the external iliac vessels distal to the inguinal ligament. At the level of the acetabulum, the artery is more lateral than the vein. Direct compression of the femoral vessels from a variety of hip positioners has been described. Retractors placed too far medially, over the anterior inferior acetabulum, may injure the common femoral vessels. Direct injury as well as intimal injury from levering the retractors has been described. Anterior osteophyte resection may also injure the femoral vessels. Intimal

*Craig J. Della Valle, MD, or the department with which he is affiliated has received research or institutional support from Zimmer, miscellaneous nonincome support, commercially derived honoraria, or other nonresearch-related funding from Zimmer, Stryker, and Smith & Nephew, and is a consultant for or an employee of Zimmer.

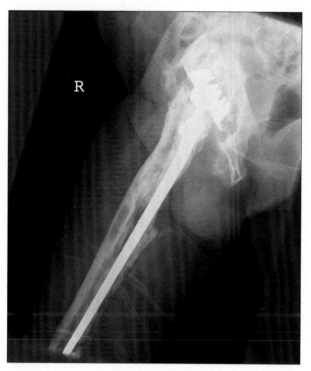

Figure 1 Preoperative radiograph showing severe femoral and acetabular bone loss with medial migration of the acetabular component.

CASE PRESENTATION 1: INTRAOPERATIVE BLEEDING

History

A 55-year-old man with cerebral palsy and a history of multiple right total hip revisions presented with increasing pain and swelling in his right hip and thigh. Upon physical examination, he had pain with range of motion of the hip and a well-healed surgical incision. The extremity was neurovascularly intact with palpable distal pulses. Radiographs showed loose components with medial migration of the acetabular component (**Figure 1**). Erythrocyte sedimentation rate and C-reactive protein levels were elevated. Aspiration of the hip demonstrated gram-negative rods. A decision was made to proceed with resection of the right hip components and spacer placement.

The Complication and Its Treatment

A posterior approach to the right hip was used. A severe inflammatory reaction about the capsule and hip components was found. The femoral component was grossly loose and was removed without difficulty. The acetabular component was also grossly loose but had fibrous attachments to the acetabulum. These attachments were carefully freed from the acetabular component. Upon removal of the cup, brisk pulsatile bleeding was encountered from the medial wall of the acetabulum. The wound was packed and a pulse was felt in the distal lower extremity. The patient remained hemodynamically stable. The packing was removed, and pulsatile bleeding was again encountered. The wound was repacked and a vascular surgery consultation was requested. Multiple units of packed red blood cells were given and the patient remained hemodynamically stable.

An attempt was made to address the source of bleeding through the acetabulum, but adequate hemostasis was not obtained. The wound was provisionally closed and the patient was placed in the supine position. The abdomen was prepared and the vascular surgeon performed a retroperitoneal approach to the pelvis. Control of the bleeding was

injury is more commonly associated with the anterolateral approaches.[1] In addition, reduction and dislocation maneuvers may result in injury to the femoral vessels.[3]

The obturator neurovascular bundle runs along the quadrilateral surface of the acetabulum. The obturator internus is interposed between the vessels and the anteroinferior acetabulum. Injury to the obturator artery or vein is less common but may occur due to retractor placement under the transverse acetabular ligament or from screws placed in the anterior inferior quadrant of the acetabulum.

Prevalence of the Complication

Calligaro and associates[4] reviewed 23,199 knee arthroplasty procedures and 9,581 THAs and found acute arterial complications in 0.13% of knee procedures and 0.17% of hip procedures. Arterial injury was diagnosed on the day of surgery in 56% of these patients; diagnosis was delayed 1 to 5 days in the remaining 44%.

gained at the common iliac artery. The external iliac artery was identified and found to be very friable, with extremely reactive tissue surrounding the vessel. A 1.5-cm longitudinal injury in the artery was identified, and an external iliac bypass graft was performed, with restoration of blood flow to the lower extremity. The retroperitoneal wound was closed and the patient was turned back to the lateral decubitus position. The wound was irrigated with pulsatile lavage. It was decided not to place an antibiotic-loaded spacer because of the degree of femoral and pelvic bone loss.

Outcome

The patient recovered uneventfully and was treated with a 6-week course of intravenous antibiotics. The wound healed and the extremity was found to be neurovascularly intact at 6-week follow-up. The patient was counseled not to undergo further surgery of the hip given the marked femoral and pelvic bone loss. At last follow-up, the patient reported occasional pain in the hip. He is a minimal in-home ambulator with a walker.

Discussion
Recognizing the Problem and High-Risk Situations

The first step in avoiding a vascular injury is to recognize possible causes and risk factors, which can be either directly related to the surgery or patient-related. Surgical causes include stretching injuries, such as from leg lengthening, or direct injury from retractor placement, component removal, or component insertion (eg, screw insertion).

Patient factors that have been shown to increase the risk of vascular injury include revision surgery; left-sided surgery (based on the relationship of the aortic bifurcation and left iliac artery); female sex; medial migration of components; and infection.[3,5] Medial (intrapelvic) migration of components, such as in the case described here, place the patient at high risk for vascular injury. Medially migrated components often adhere to the pelvic contents, such as the iliac vessels. Forceful removal of the components from the lateral hip wound may tear the adherent vessel. Intrapelvic cement is often difficult and dangerous to remove using traditional revision exposures; if removal is necessary (such as in the case of an infection), a retroperitoneal approach to the hip may be required. Cement that has migrated slowly into the pelvis is typically less problematic than cement that has been intrapelvic from the time of its polymerization, as polymerizing cement may adhere to vessel walls. During routine revision procedures, it is often not necessary to remove the intrapelvic cement unless infection is present.

Intrapelvic migration of the acetabular component has also been found to be frequently associated with periprosthetic infection. Stiehl[5] has reported that infection was present in half of the patients with severe intrapelvic component migration. Infected periprosthetic tissue may adhere to the acetabular component and make removal more dangerous. This infected tissue is often more friable and prone to a tearing or shearing vessel injury.

Acute Management of Uncontrolled Intraoperative Bleeding

Uncontrolled intraoperative bleeding is uncommon during THA; when it does occur, however, it must be controlled immediately. It is important to be aware of the fact that retroperitoneal or intrapelvic bleeding may not be visualized in the surgical field; a sudden drop in blood pressure and tachycardia following a risky maneuver may be the first sign of a vascular injury. If a major vessel injury is suspected, a vascular surgeon should be consulted intraoperatively. If the source of bleeding is identified but cannot be stopped, direct pressure may be applied to the area of the bleeding. If the source cannot be identified, the wound should be packed. Aggressive volume replacement, including packed red blood cells and relevant blood products, should be started immediately.

If the patient remains hemodynamically unstable or an intrapelvic vascular injury is suspected, the wound should be closed quickly and the patient positioned for laparotomy by a vascular or general surgeon. Vessel repair and/or embolization is often performed by the consulting vascular surgeon.

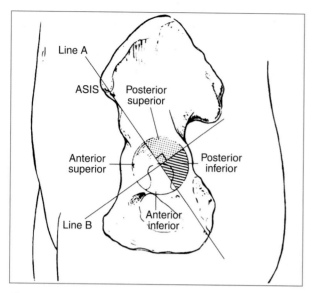

Figure 2 Quadrant system for safe placement of acetabular screws. ASIS = anterior superior iliac spine. (Reproduced with permission from Wasielewski RC, Cooperstein LA, Kruger MP, Rubash HE: Acetabular anatomy and the transacetabular fixation of screws in total hip arthroplasty. *J Bone Joint Surg Am* 1990;72:501-508.)

Preventing Vascular Injury
Preoperative Evaluation

A thorough preoperative evaluation should be performed in conjunction with a vascular or general surgeon in all patients with medially migrated acetabular components. A contrast-enhanced CT scan is often helpful to identify the location of the acetabular component in relationship to vital structures such as arteries and veins.[6] Additional studies such as angiograms or cystograms may be necessary. Components that are close to vascular structures may be removed with an intrapelvic or retroperitoneal approach performed by a general or vascular surgeon.[7-9]

Screw Placement

Wasielewski and associates[10] have described a quadrant system for placement of acetabular screws. The acetabulum is divided into anterior and posterior halves by a line drawn from the anterior superior iliac spine (ASIS) to bisect the acetabulum.

Another line is drawn perpendicular to this line (**Figure 2**). These two lines create four quadrants. The external iliac vessels are at risk in the anterior superior quadrant, and the obturator vessels are at risk in the anterior inferior quadrant. The safest zone is the posterior superior quadrant. This quadrant contains the greatest bone depth, so 35-mm screws may be used. However, screws longer than this may injure the sciatic nerve or superior gluteal artery. The posterior inferior quadrant is the next safest. However, the bone is not as thick in this quadrant, so screws >25 mm should be avoided. The inferior gluteal and internal pudendal vessels are at risk in this quadrant. If screws are used in the anterior quadrants, unicortical fixation should be considered.

In a cadaveric study of acetabular reconstruction cages, Lavernia and associates[11] described a "safe zone" for screw locations and depths. The authors recommended 15-mm screws for the superior flange and 25-mm screws for the posterior rim. In addition, if a high hip center is used, only the peripheral half of the posterior quadrant is safe for screw placement.[12]

CASE PRESENTATION 2: POSTOPERATIVE PERIPHERAL VASCULAR COMPROMISE
History

A 77-year-old man presented with severe hip pain secondary to degenerative arthritis. Medical comorbidities included diabetes mellitus, coronary artery disease, congestive heart failure, atrial fibrillation, hypertension, prostate cancer, and peripheral vascular disease. Relevant surgical history included an aortobifemoral bypass 10 years prior to presentation, with a graft revision 3 years later. Physical examination revealed a painful and restricted range of motion of the right hip with palpable pedal pulses.

The Complication and Its Treatment

A right THA was performed through a posterior approach; the surgery was uneventful. Warfarin prophylaxis was administered. On the evening of the third postoperative day, the patient presented with increasingly severe lower right extremity pain that was unresponsive to pain medications. On physical examination, distal pulses were absent and the distal lower extremity was cooler than the contralateral limb. The patient also had loss of active dorsiflexion of the ankle and great toe, along with decreased sensation on the dorsum of the foot.

A vascular surgeon was consulted and the patient was taken emergently to the operating room. A clot was found in the aortobifemoral graft. A thrombectomy was attempted and failed. A revision of the aortobifemoral graft was performed along with fasciotomies of the lower leg.

Outcome

The perioperative course was complicated by chronic renal failure, respiratory failure requiring extended intubation, and a pneumothorax requiring a chest tube. Delirium persisted following eventual extubation. The patient was discharged to a rehabilitation center on postoperative day 25.

Discussion

Recognizing the Problem and High-Risk Situations

Patients with absent or diminished pulses, a history of peripheral vascular disease, or previous bypass or revascularization procedures are at increased risk for vascular complications after THA. In addition, patients with comorbidities (eg, diabetes mellitus, coronary artery disease) that are associated with peripheral vascular disease also may be at increased risk. Caution must be exercised in patients with diabetes or peripheral vascular disease because Doppler studies such as the ankle-brachial index may be inaccurate in these patients.[13] Arterial calcification results in noncompressibility and noncompliance of the vessels, yielding a falsely normal study.[14]

Acute Management

Vascular compromise diagnosed postoperatively should be considered a surgical emergency. Presentation may vary from an obvious dysvascular limb to subtle findings of pain, neurologic changes, or compartment syndrome. Urgent vascular assessment is necessary, and a vascular

surgical consultation should not be delayed. If the limb appears compromised, the patient should be taken immediately to the operating room and assessed by a vascular surgeon. If the limb appears compromised but viable, noninvasive or invasive (angiographic) evaluation may be necessary. If limb viability is threatened, however, surgery should not be delayed to obtain imaging studies. The patient should proceed to the operating room without delay to limit the ischemic time to the limb.

Preventing Vascular Injury in Patients With Preexisting Vascular Disease

Patients with a history of peripheral vascular disease should undergo preoperative testing and evaluation by a vascular surgeon. Workup may include noninvasive studies (ultrasound or duplex scan) or an arteriogram. In this case, the patient had a previous aortobifemoral bypass graft. Trousdale and associates[15] have postulated that the posterior surgical approach with the limb in a flexed, adducted, internally rotated position during femoral preparation may put these types of grafts at risk. Extreme positions of the limb should be minimized as much as possible.[16]

STRATEGIES TO MINIMIZE COMMON COMPLICATIONS

Intraoperative Vascular Injury

Prevention of intraoperative vascular injury begins with appropriate preoperative planning, especially during revision surgery. Prior surgical reports should be reviewed to ascertain if there was a previous vascular injury or difficulty. If a medially migrated acetabular component is being revised, preoperative CT scans may be necessary, as previously discussed. Gentle surgical technique should be used. Forceful dislocation of the native hip or previous implants should be avoided because vascular complications from shearing or tearing of the vessels have been described. Anterior retractors should be placed carefully. Retractors should be placed directly on bone, using care to avoid soft-tissue (which may contain an artery or vein) impingement. It is best to place the anterior acetabular retractors with the hip in a flexed position as this takes tension off the femoral neurovascular bundle. In addition, assistants holding the anterior retractors should be monitored for overzealous retraction. During revision surgery, assessment of the remaining acetabular anatomy is crucial before placing retractors. Forceful removal of medially migrated components, even if grossly loose, should be avoided because soft-tissue attachment to the components and vascular structures may be present. Aggressive reaming through the medial wall should be avoided. Careful screw insertion with knowledge of the quadrant system and accurate measurement of screw lengths are imperative.

Patients With Preexisting Vascular Disease

When planning hip surgery in patients with preexisting vascular disease, a preoperative workup may be indicated. Patients with known severe vascular disease or absent pulses should have a preoperative consultation with a vascular surgeon. Noninvasive studies or angiograms may be necessary. Preoperative angioplasty, stenting, or vascular bypass may be necessary. Intraoperatively, extremes of rotation and adduction should be avoided or minimized to reduce the shearing of the vascular structures.

SUMMARY

The incidence of vascular injury after THA is low, but when it does occur, it can be devastating to the patient. Vigilant preoperative evaluation combined with precise surgical technique is imperative. Vascular injuries may occur at any time during the surgical procedure, and high-risk scenarios should be considered. If vascular injury does occur, it should be addressed meticulously and quickly with the aid of a vascular surgeon if necessary. If prolonged limb ischemia occurs, prophylactic lower extremity fasciotomy is recommended.

REFERENCES

1. Wasielewski RC, Crossett LS, Rubash HE: Neural and vascular injury in total hip arthroplasty. *Orthop Clin North Am* 1992;23:219-235.

2. Nachbur B, Meyer RP, Verkkala K, Zurcher R: The mechanisms of severe arterial injury in surgery of the hip joint. *Clin Orthop Relat Res* 1979;141: 122-133.

3. Shoenfeld NA, Stuchin SA, Pearl R, Haveson S: The management of vascular injuries associated with total hip arthroplasty. *J Vasc Surg* 1990;11:549-555.

4. Calligaro KD, Dougherty MJ, Ryan S, Booth RE: Acute arterial complications associated with total hip and knee arthroplasty. *J Vasc Surg* 2003;38:1170-1177.

5. Stiehl JB: Acetabular prosthetic protrusion and sepsis: Case report and review of the literature. *J Arthroplasty* 2007;22: 283-288.

6. Fehring TK, Guilford WB, Baron J: Assessment of intrapelvic cement and screws in revision total hip arthroplasty. *J Arthroplasty* 1992;7:509-518.

7. Petrera P, Trakru S, Mehta S, Steed D, Towers JD, Rubash HE: Revision total hip arthroplasty with a retroperitoneal approach to the iliac vessels. *J Arthroplasty* 1996;11: 704-708.

8. Eftekhar NS, Nercessian O: Intrapelvic migration of total hip prostheses: Operative treatment. *J Bone Joint Surg Am* 1989;71:1480-1486.

9. al-Salman M, Taylor DC, Beauchamp CP, Duncan CP: Prevention of vascular injuries in revision total hip replacement. *Can J Surg* 1992;35:261-264.

10. Wasielewski RC, Cooperstein LA, Kruger MP, Rubash HE: Acetabular anatomy and the transacetabular fixation of screws in total hip arthroplasty. *J Bone Joint Surg Am* 1990; 72:501-508.

11. Lavernia CJ, Cook CC, Hernandez RA, Sierra RJ, Rossi MD: Neurovascular injuries in acetabular reconstruction cage surgery: An anatomical study. *J Arthroplasty* 2007;22:124-132.

12. Wasielewski RC, Galat DD, Sheridan KC, Rubash HE: Acetabular anatomy and transacetabular screw fixation at the high hip center. *Clin Orthop Relat Res* 2005;438:171-176.

13. Goss DE, de Trafford J, Roberts VC, Flynn MD, Edmonds ME, Watkins PJ: Raised ankle/ brachial pressure index in insulin-treated diabetic patients. *Diabet Med* 1989;6:576-578.

14. Wyss CR, Harrington RM, Burgess EM, Matsen FA III: Transcutaneous oxygen tension as a predictor of success after an amputation. *J Bone Joint Surg Am* 1988;70:203-207.

15. Trousdale RT, Donnelly RS, Hallett JW: Thrombosis of an aortobifemoral bypass graft after total hip arthroplasty. *J Arthroplasty* 1999;14:386-390.

16. Cameron HU: Hip surgery in aortofemoral bypass patients. *Orthop Rev* 1988;17:195-197.

Chapter 3

PERIPROSTHETIC FRACTURE

Brett Levine, MD, MS
*Craig J. Della Valle, MD

Periprosthetic fracture after total hip arthroplasty (THA) is an increasingly common complication that may occur intraoperatively or postoperatively. Intraoperative fractures of the femur have been reported to occur in 0.3% to 6.3% of cases, varying based on femoral component fixation (cemented versus cementless).[1-6] The incidence of postoperative fractures of the femur ranges from 0.1% to 2.1%.[1,3,7] The rising incidence of these fractures and their complex management have made them the focus of increasing study.

CASE PRESENTATION 1: NONDISPLACED INTRAOPERATIVE FRACTURE OF THE FEMUR

History

A 51-year-old woman with a history of rheumatoid arthritis presented with progressively worsening left hip pain refractory to nonsteroidal anti-inflammatory drugs (NSAIDs), corticosteroid injections, and activity modification. She was electively scheduled for a left THA.

A tapered, proximally coated femoral implant was chosen intraoperatively. Reaming and broaching were completed without complication. During impaction of the final implant, excellent purchase was obtained proximally with rigid rotational and axial stability. On further inspection, however, a nondisplaced fracture of the femoral neck extending distally just proximal to the lesser trochanter was noted.

Management

The implant had rotational and axial stability, so it was decided that the femoral component could be retained, and a cable was placed distal to the

*Craig Della Valle, MD, or the department with which he is affiliated has received research or institutional support from Zimmer, miscellaneous nonincome support, commercially derived honoraria, or other nonresearch-related funding from Zimmer, Stryker, and Smith & Nephew, and is a consultant for or employee of Zimmer.

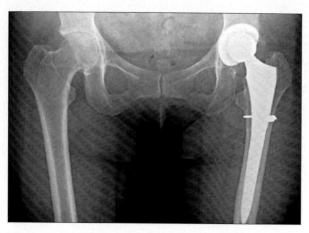

Figure 1 A 51-year-old woman with a history of rheumatoid arthritis sustained an intraoperative fracture of the proximal femur. The fracture was treated with retention of the implant and cable fixation. AP radiograph obtained at 2-year follow-up shows a well-fixed femoral component.

lesser trochanter to prevent fracture propagation. The patient was then placed on restricted weight bearing (foot-flat) for the next 6 weeks. Progression to full weight bearing was allowed over the following 6 weeks, to allow unassisted ambulation at 3 months.

Outcome

At 3 months, the patient was able to ambulate more than five blocks without assistive devices and without pain. She participated in physical therapy, and by 6 months, she was able to ambulate unlimited distances without pain, limitations, or a limp. She navigated stairs in a reciprocating fashion without using the railing and returned to work without restrictions. At 2 years from the index procedure, the patient has not had any further complications, and radiographs demonstrate a stable implant (**Figure 1**).

Discussion

Recognizing the Problem and High-Risk Situations

The first step in preventing intraoperative fractures of the femur during THA is to identify patients who are at high risk for this complication. Risk factors can be divided into two categories—host characteristics and technique-related factors.

Host Characteristics

Risk factors for intraoperative periprosthetic fractures of the femur include female sex, revision surgery, increased bone fragility (osteoporosis), and inflammatory arthritis.[4,5] Patients with a deformity (congenital or acquired) of the proximal femur or femoral shaft are at a higher risk for intraoperative fracture. Berend and associates[8] found higher fracture rates in patients undergoing THA for conditions other than osteoarthritis.

Technique-Related Factors

Surgical technique plays a crucial role in the prevalence of intraoperative periprosthetic fractures of the femur. Varying rates of fracture have been reported with techniques such as cemented versus cementless femoral components, different surgical approaches, and minimally or less invasive surgical exposures.[9] The modern trend toward using cementless femoral components increases the risk and incidence of intraoperative fractures of the femur[10] because they require a tight press-fit, which is not imperative for cemented fixation.[11] Although preoperative templating is a helpful guide in using appropriate sized implants, fracture may occur at any point during preparation of the femoral canal, as well as with seating of the final prosthesis. Attention to detail during reaming and broaching can minimize technical errors and the risk of intraoperative fracture. When trial implants are several sizes larger or smaller than the preoperative template, typically femoral canal preparation has gone awry.

Intraoperative fracture location can vary based on the geometry and design of the selected femoral implant. Stems that rely on distal fixation are more likely to be associated with fractures at the stem tip, whereas proximal fixation components are more likely to be associated with fractures around the level of the greater and lesser trochanters. Familiarity with inserting these implants gives the surgeon the tactile feel for when the risk for fracture is increasing. Intraoperative fractures may also occur at the time of trial or final reduction of the hip, when the rotational stresses at the prosthetic tip may lead to spiral fracture of the femoral shaft (**Figure 2**).

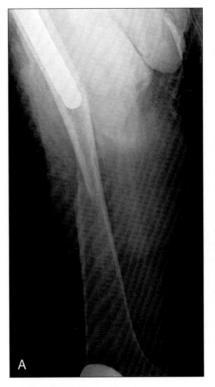 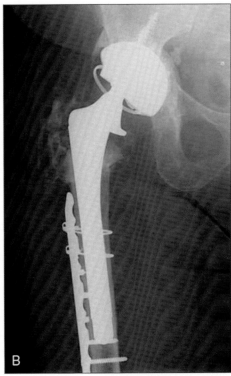 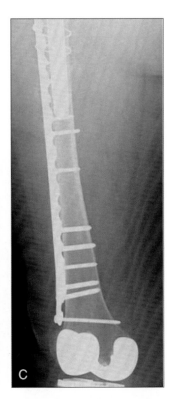

Figure 2 Radiographs of an intraoperative fracture of the femur that occurred during the final reduction of a revision THA. **A,** Intraoperative radiograph shows a spiral fracture at the tip of the femoral stem. **B,** AP radiograph of the proximal femur at 3-month follow-up. **C,** AP view shows the distal extent of the fixation at 3-month follow-up.

Use of an anterolateral approach for THA also has been reported to increase the risk of intraoperative fracture.[9] Berend and Bertrand[9] postulate that anatomic factors such as femoral neck angle and offset, bone density, and metaphyseal geometry may explain the increased risk associated with the anterolateral approach. Similarly, minimally and less invasive surgical approaches have been reported to have higher incidences of intraoperative fractures of the femur.[9] The lack of visualization and technical difficulty ("learning curve") of these approaches has been accompanied by an increased incidence of fracture.[12-14]

Greidanus and associates[15] have described the Vancouver classification for intra-operative periprosthetic fractures of the femur. The classification is shown in **Table 1.**

Intraoperative Fractures

Intraoperative fractures of the femur occur in roughly 3.5% of primary cementless THAs and in 0.4% of cemented THAs.[16] Proximal fractures of the femur occurring during THA often may be treated with retention of the femoral prosthesis and cerclage wiring or cabling of the fracture, when axial and torsional stability are maintained.[3,8] Fracture healing and implant survival occur at high rates with standard length implants and cabling or wiring of the fracture (**Figure 1**). When torsional and/or axial stability cannot be maintained despite fixation of the fracture, then conversion to a longer stem with distal fixation is required.[4,5,9,17] **Figure 3** shows a case in which a tapered, proximally coated implant was planned. During preparation of the femoral canal, a

TABLE 1 Vancouver Classification for Intraoperative Periprosthetic Fractures of the Femur

Type	Location	Characteristics
A1	Proximal metaphysis	Cortical perforation
A2	Proximal metaphysis	Nondisplaced crack
A3	Proximal metaphysis	Unstable fracture
B1	Diaphysis	Cortical perforation
B2	Diaphysis	Nondisplaced crack
B3	Diaphysis	Displaced fracture
C1	Distal diaphysis/metaphysis	Cortical perforation
C2	Distal diaphysis/metaphysis	Nondisplaced crack extending into the distal metaphysis
C3	Distal diaphysis/metaphysis	Displaced distal fracture

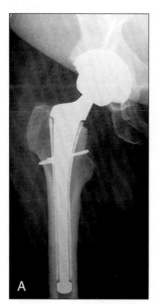
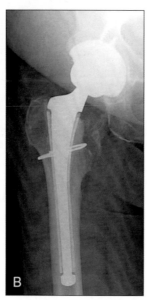

Figure 3 AP radiographs of a hip that sustained an intraoperative fracture of the proximal femur during implantation of a proximally tapered prosthesis. The fracture compromised the stability of the implant, which thus was converted to a distally fixed stem with cabling of the fracture. **A,** Radiograph of the hip immediately after conversion to the distally fixed stem. **B,** At 3-month follow-up, the implant was stable and there were no signs of fracture propagation.

fracture of the femoral neck was found and a longer stem with distal fixation was substituted; the fracture was treated with a cerclage wire.

Middle-region fractures typically occur during a difficult exposure or with bone preparation. Patients with weak bone (prior surgery, poor bone quality, etc), protrusio acetabuli, or soft-tissue contractures are at risk for intraoperative fractures of the femur during surgical exposure. In situ femoral neck or trochanteric osteotomy may facilitate exposure and avoid undue stress on the middle region of the proximal femur.[16]

Fractures distal to the femoral stem are often not recognized intraoperatively and typically do not compromise fixation of the implant. These fractures typically occur when the tip of a straight stem impacts the bow of the femur.[4,16] When these fractures are nondisplaced, limited weight bearing for 6 weeks is usually sufficient for fracture healing without further repercussion. In the case of a displaced fracture or unstable implant, reoperation to stabilize the fracture and/or the implant is indicated.[3,17]

Because of the complex, costly, and high-risk nature of treating periprosthetic fractures of the femur, every effort should be made to prevent such fractures.[18] The risk of an intraoperative fracture can be decreased by attention to detail during femoral canal preparation and insertion of the final implant. Adequate exposure is extremely important, as is the avoidance of eccentric reaming of the femoral canal.[18] During broaching of the femur, it is important to ensure that the broach advances with progressive mallet blows; if it does not, the chances of fracture are high. Similarly, if the implant advances past the level of the final broach, a periprosthetic fracture should be assumed and either searched for visually or on an intraoperative radiograph. Finally, when inserting a diaphyseal-engaging stem, it is important to recognize that the size listed on the implant box may vary from the size of the actual implant second-

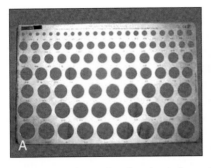
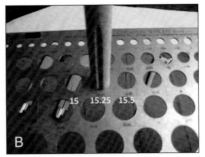
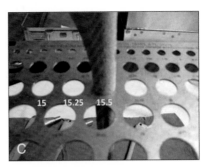

Figure 4 Measuring implant size using a hole gauge. **A,** Hole gauge used to measure fully coated implants. **B** and **C,** A size 15 stem is trialed through the hole gauge. As a result of the sintering process, this stem measures just over 15.25 mm in diameter.

ary to variability in the sintering process. Thus, we recommend measuring the size of the implant using a hole gauge (**Figure 4**) to ensure that the canal is underreamed by an appropriate amount (0.25 to 0.5 mm). Prophylactic cabling or wiring of the femur can be a useful technique in preventing fracture propagation if one has already occurred.

CASE PRESENTATION 2: EARLY POSTOPERATIVE FRACTURE OF THE FEMUR

History

A 56-year-old woman (5'11" tall, approximately 360 lb; body mass index = 50) presented 4 weeks after a primary THA with a double-tapered, proximally coated, cementless femoral stem and cementless acetabular component. She progressed well initially following surgery, but then noted inability to bear weight on the extremity following a fall from a standing height.

Radiographs taken after the fall showed a displaced fracture of the proximal femur. The femoral and acetabular components were in place, but subsidence of the tapered femoral component was evident (**Figure 5, A**).

Management

The patient was admitted to the hospital and evaluated preoperatively for revision surgery. During the

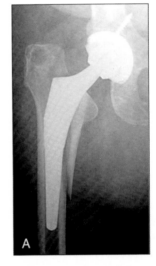
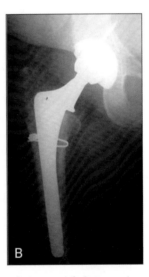

Figure 5 Early postoperative fracture of the proximal femur in a 56-year-old woman. **A,** AP radiograph demonstrates a Vancouver type B2 fracture, possibly secondary to an unrecognized intraoperative fracture. The original surgery was via a minimally invasive Watson-Jones approach. **B,** AP radiograph obtained after revision surgery with conversion to a distal fixation device and cabling of the fracture.

procedure, the loose femoral component was removed and a diaphyseal-engaging stem was placed. A cerclage cable was placed proximally around the femur to reduce the fracture.

The patient was placed on touch-down weight bearing for 6 weeks, followed by progressive weight bearing with an assistive device for the next 6 weeks. She was allowed to discontinue use of an assistive device at 3 months.

Outcome

The fracture healed uneventfully and the stem had osseointegrated at latest follow-up (**Figure 5, B**).

Discussion

Recognizing the Problem and High-Risk Situations

The incidence of early postoperative periprosthetic fractures of the femur is difficult to accurately determine because many fractures may occur intraoperatively. The overall rate of postoperative periprosthetic fractures for primary THA has been reported to be between 0.1% and 2.1%.[1,3,7] Most early fractures are secondary to unrecognized intraoperative fractures or are associated with iatrogenic defects produced during preparation of the femoral canal (cortical perforation or eccentric reaming).[16,19,20] With minimally invasive techniques being used more frequently, these intraoperative fractures may increasingly go unrecognized during the surgical procedure and lead to an increase in reported early postoperative periprosthetic fractures.[12-14] In the revision setting, early fracture is often related to areas of cement and/or hardware removal, creating a stress riser in the early postoperative period. It is important to recognize these potential areas that may serve as stress risers and treat them with bone graft, order protected weight bearing, or bypass them with a longer femoral stem (twice the bone diameter).[1,3,16,17] Careful femoral canal preparation, a low threshold for supplemental fixation, and a thorough review of postoperative radiographs may afford early detection of these risk factors and help prevent a new fracture or propagation of an intraoperative fracture.

Treatment Options

The main goals in treating these early periprosthetic fractures of the femur are fracture union and maintenance of a stable prosthesis. Historically, a high rate of complications has been associated with periprosthetic fractures of the femur, with Beals and Tower[21] reporting 41% and 33% complications relating to either the fracture or the arthroplasty, respectively. Treatment is similar to that described above for intraoperative fractures. Proximal fractures are often longitudinal splits of the femoral neck and do not disrupt the stability of the implant. These fractures may be treated with modified weight bearing until the fracture is healed. If the stability of the implant is compromised or the fracture extends, leading to implant subsidence, then revision to a long-stem distally engaging implant should be performed with cable/wire fixation of the fracture.

Middle-region fractures typically have a high union rate and may be treated nonsurgically if the implant remains stable.[16] Distal fractures at the tip of the stem may be treated nonsurgically if the implant remains stable and the fracture is nondisplaced (**Figure 6**). Historically these patients were treated with a spica cast with excellent results.[4] Patients today typically will not tolerate spica casting; therefore, activity modification is the usual treatment for nondisplaced and minimally displaced fractures. However, if the fracture is displaced or propagation is noted on early postoperative radiographs, then surgical revision and fracture stabilization are recommended.[4]

Early periprosthetic fractures with an unstable implant require revision to a distally fixed implant with fixation of the fracture using cables/wires, a plate, or cortical onlay strut allograft fixation.[3,20] Ideally the femoral prosthesis should bypass the distal extent of the fracture by at least two cortical diameters. A study in canine femora has shown that bypassing a cortical penetration by two cortical diameters increases the femoral strength to 84% of that of the contralateral femur.[22] Proximally porous-coated stems have not had success in treating these fractures and should be avoided in such situations.[1,20]

Extensively coated or fluted long-stem devices gain distal fixation and provide torsional stability to the distal fragment. Excellent results have been reported using these devices in revision THA, with cortical strut grafts providing additional torsional and bending stability when needed.[1,20,23,24] Springer and associates[25] found a 0% nonunion rate and better results with extensively coated stems used in revision THA for periprosthetic fracture. For optimal stability and

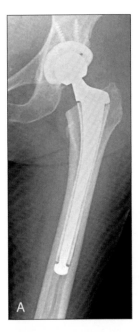
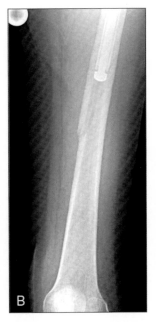
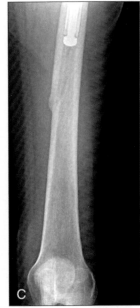

Figure 6 Early postoperative fracture of the middle femur. **A,** AP radiograph shows minimally displaced fracture at the tip of the fully coated stem. Treatment was with protected weight bearing. **B,** AP view taken at 3-month follow-up. **C,** AP weight-bearing view taken at 6-month follow-up shows a healed fracture.

long-term success, it is recommended that a minimum of 4 to 6 cm of intimate isthmal fixation be achieved when using extensively coated femoral components.[20] In cases of early periprosthetic fractures, bone quality is often less of a concern because stress-shielding, osteolysis, and implant loosening are not likely to have occurred before the fracture. Therefore, we recommend conversion to an extensively coated implant when these early fractures do occur with loss of fixation of the femoral component.

CASE PRESENTATION 3: LATE POSTOPERATIVE FRACTURE OF THE FEMUR

History

A 72-year-old woman presented to the emergency department after a fall from a standing height. She reported right thigh and hip pain. She had a history of a hybrid THA performed several years before the fall. After further questioning, the patient reported approximately 3 weeks of dull thigh pain before the fall.

Radiographs taken in the emergency department revealed a hybrid THA with a stable acetabular component and a fracture at the tip of the femoral component. The fracture had disrupted the cement mantle, and the femoral component was loose (**Figure 7, *A***).

Management

The patient underwent revision surgery with an extended trochanteric osteotomy (ETO) to assist in cement removal. The osteotomy was made to the level of the fracture where it meets the lateral femoral cortex. An 8-in, cementless, diaphysis-engaging femoral component was inserted, and the fracture/osteotomy was approximated using cerclage cables (**Figure 7, *B***).

The patient was placed on touch-down weight bearing for 6 weeks, followed by progression to full weight bearing with an assistive device by 3 months. Unassisted ambulation was allowed at 3 months. Active abduction was restricted for 6 weeks and resisted abduction for 12 weeks.

Outcome

The fracture and osteotomy healed uneventfully, and the patient returned to unassisted ambulation by 4 months. Radiographs showed evidence of osseoin-

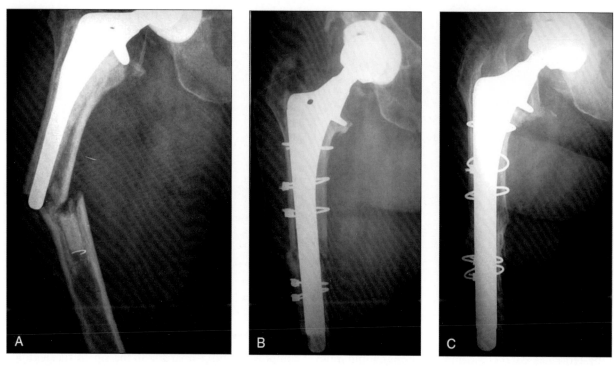

Figure 7 Late postoperative fracture of the femur in a 72-year-old woman. **A,** AP radiograph demonstrates a Vancouver type B2 fracture. **B,** AP radiograph obtained after an extended trochanteric osteotomy was used for implant/cement extraction. **C,** AP radiograph obtained at latest follow-up shows a healed fracture and osseointegrated femoral stem.

tegration and a well-fixed femoral component (**Figure 7, C**).

Discussion

Recognizing the Problem and High-Risk Situations

In contrast to early periprosthetic fractures, late fractures typically occur in the setting of loose femoral components, osteolytic lesions, and osteoporotic bone. Patients who are elderly, female, and/or have had indwelling prostheses for many years are at higher risk for late periprosthetic fractures of the femur. Such fractures are often the result of low-energy injuries such as a fall from a standing height. It has been reported that in up to 50% of periprosthetic fractures of the femur, insidious thigh pain precedes the traumatic event leading to fracture.[1] The prevalence of these fractures is clearly on the rise as there is a greater proportion of the population at risk and an increasing number of THAs and revision THAs being performed each year. Recent studies have found 1-year mortality rates for periprosthetic fractures of the femur to be similar to those of patients with a hip fracture (11% and 16.5%, respectively).[26] The probability of death as a result of the fracture for individuals 80 years of age or older is 3.9% for men and 2.2% for women.[27] The complex treatment required for these fractures and their rising prevalence present a serious burden to the healthcare system and revision surgeons of the future. However, improved surveillance with serial radiographs and recognizing the appropriate risk factors may aid in preventing periprosthetic femur factures.

Fracture location, prosthesis stability, bone quality, patient age, and medical comorbidities all play a role in determining treatment options. The Vancouver classification most accurately accounts for these factors and is the most widely accepted classification system for periprosthetic fractures of the femur.[11] Implant stability and periprosthetic bone quality/quantity are paramount in determining the appropriate treatment. A loose implant requires revision, and displaced fractures associated with a well-fixed implant necessitate open reduction and internal fixation.[11,28] The discussion below highlights the Vancouver classification and treatment options for each fracture type.

Vancouver Classification

Type A Fractures

Vancouver type A involves a fracture of the proximal femur within the trochanteric region with a stable femoral component. Type A fractures are subdivided into two categories, those involving the lesser trochanter (AL) and those involving the greater trochanter (AG).[15] Fractures of the lesser trochanter often can be treated nonsurgically; however, an isolated fracture of the lesser trochanter should raise suspicion of the possibility of a pathologic etiology of the fracture. Fractures of the greater trochanter may be associated with avulsion of the abductor musculature, secondary to weakening of the bone from osteolysis, stress-shielding, or trauma. Displaced fractures of the greater trochanter may be treated with open reduction and internal fixation. Cable plates, cable grips (claws), or cerclage wiring can be used for fixation; however, wear-related fractures of the greater trochanter also require acetabular revision (either liner exchange or full revision).[3] Wang and associates[29] reported successful treatment of 18 out of 19 greater trochanter fractures associated with osteolytic lesions using monofilament stainless-steel cerclage wire in a figure-of-8 pattern. The average time to fracture union was 5 months. When managing these fractures, tension on the repair should be minimal.

Type B1 Fracture

A Vancouver type B1 fracture originates at the tip or just distal to the stem without compromising the stability of the femoral component. Nonsurgical management of these fractures has had disappointing results, with high rates of malunion, nonunion, and implant loosening.[3] Typically, open reduction and

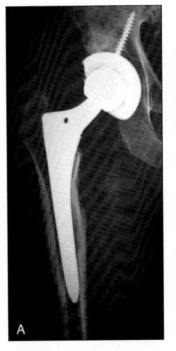
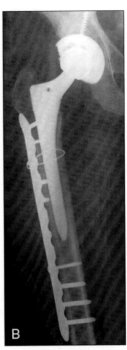

Figure 8 AP radiographs of a Vancouver type B1 periprosthetic fracture that occurred from a fall from standing. **A,** Preoperative radiograph. **B,** Surgical fixation was achieved using a long locking compression plate.

internal fixation is the treatment of choice in these cases (**Figure 8**). Several options exist in treating these fractures, including locked femoral plating, cable plates, strut allograft fixation, or a combination of these modalities. Dennis and associates[30] reviewed five options for fixation of a periprosthetic fracture of the femur to determine overall construct stability. The five fixation options were plate and cables, plate with proximal cables and distal bicortical screws, plate with proximal unicortical screws and distal bicortical screws, plate with proximal cables and unicortical screws and distal bicortical screws, and two allograft struts fixed with cables. The constructs using plate fixation with proximal cables and/or unicortical screws with distal bicortical screw fixation were significantly more stable in axial compression, lateral bending, and torsional loading compared to the other three tested options.[30]

In 2002, Haddad and associates[31] reported on 40 periprosthetic fractures treated with cortical onlay allografts with or without concomitant plate fixation. In this study, 98% of the fractures healed, leading the authors to conclude that cortical strut allografts used alone or in combination with plate fixation can lead to a high rate of fracture union, satisfactory alignment, and increased femoral bone stock at short-term follow-up.[31] However, concerns with the use of strut allografts (ie, expense, disease transmission, soft-tissue stripping during application, and weakening during incorporation) prompted a study by Old and associates[32] using broad metal (4 locking and 15 standard) plates without bone graft for fixation of Vancouver type B1 fractures. They reported fracture healing in 18 out of 19 cases, with an average time to weight bearing of 10 weeks. Despite some reports of good results, there have been recent reports with a lower rate of union, and the current literature reports a range of 33% to 100% rates of fracture healing in treating Vancouver type B1 injuries.[33] Buttaro and associates[33] reported failure of fixation in 6 out of 14 (43%) cases using a locked compression plate technique. In four of these six failures, the authors elected to not use supplemental cortical struts. Despite the proven strength of locked plating, they report a high rate of complications using this technique in Vancouver type B1 fractures with well-fixed cemented implants.

Despite some mixed results, it is generally agreed that Vancouver type B1 periprosthetic fractures of the femur require surgical management (either revision arthroplasty or internal fixation). The most important factors in determining the long-term success in treating these difficult cases include proper classification of the fracture (making sure the stem is not loose), implant alignment (femoral stems in varus are associated with high rates of plate failure and implant loosening), preservation of the periosteal blood supply of the femur, and adequate protection of potential stress risers.[3] Meticulous surgical technique and close attention to these aforementioned factors for long-term success can minimize postoperative complications and enhance fracture healing and clinical results.

Type B2 Fracture

Vancouver type B2 involves a fracture around the tip of the femoral stem with a loose femoral component and reasonable quality bone remaining proximally.

The loose femoral component requires revision surgery, which can be performed using extensively coated femoral stems; modular tapered stems; allograft-prosthetic composites; or megaprostheses.[3,34] Implant choices for revision surgery are based on the Paprosky classification of the femur.[35] Proximal fixation stems have been reported to have a low level of success and high early loosening rates.[1] In the presence of a Paprosky type IIIA femoral defect, a cylindrical, diaphyseal-engaging implant can be used safely as long as 4 cm of intact femoral isthmus is available for distal fixation. In type IIIB defects, the diaphysis remains supportive but less than 4 cm of isthmus is available for distal fixation, and distal-engaging, modular tapered stems are favored.[35] Regardless of the implant selected, the fracture should be bypassed by at least two cortical diameters. Preoperative templating can be helpful in these cases and guide the appropriate implant selection and required allografts.

In cases of a loose cemented femoral implant, varus remodeling, or need for better exposure, an ETO can be useful. Osteotomy length is based on the level of the fracture at the lateral femoral cortex. A carefully planned and executed osteotomy allows relative ease of insertion of the femoral component, removal of a well-fixed cement mantle, and correction of any acquired deformities of the proximal femur without compromise of fracture healing and outcome.[36] A vital step in performing a successful ETO in the setting of a periprosthetic fracture is to place a cable/wire just distal to the osteotomy site before reaming the femoral canal. Without protection of the cortical tube distally, it is possible that reaming and/or insertion of the final implant may cause propagation of the fracture/osteotomy into the distal fragment. Ko and associates[37] reported on 14 revision THAs using a cementless conical femoral stem with a transfemoral approach through the fracture site. The 12 patients available at 58.5 months' follow-up were found to have healed fractures and stable femoral stems. Similarly, Mulay and associates[36] reported on 24 patients using a transfemoral approach to treat Vancouver B2 and B3 periprosthetic fractures of the femur; 91% of the fractures went on to union with a stable femoral implant at latest follow-up.

Type B3 Fracture

Vancouver type B3 fractures occur around the femoral stem and are associated with femoral component loosening and poor quality bone stock. A tapered implant is often required because the isthmal bone of the femur is compromised and less than 4 cm of isthmal fixation is available. Modular and nonmodular rough-surfaced tapered implants have been used successfully in these cases.[36-38] Berry[38] reported on eight Vancouver type B3 fractures treated with a long, modular, fluted, tapered cementless stem. Of the seven patients available at latest follow-up, all had achieved fracture union with stable femoral components, and all returned to ambulate with minimal thigh pain. As with type B2 fractures, use of an ETO can be helpful for exposure, cement removal, femoral implant insertion, and deformity correction.

In cases of extremely poor bone stock and lower-demand patients, megaprostheses and allograft-prosthetic composites (APCs) can also be used. Difficulty in gaining femoral stem stability while simultaneously achieving fracture fixation in the absence of proximal femoral bone support has led to the use of APCs and proximal femoral replacements. Springer and associates[25] reported on 18 cases in which an APC (14 cases) or a proximal femoral replacement (4 cases) were used to treat periprosthetic fractures of the femur. Seven of these 18 cases (39%) went on to loosening (6 aseptic and 1 septic) at an average of 69 months. Klein and associates[39] specifically studied the use of a modular proximal femoral replacement in treating periprosthetic fractures of the femur. Twenty-one patients were included in their study at an average 3.2-year follow-up. Twenty patients retained their ability to ambulate and reported minimal or no postoperative pain. Postoperative complications included persistent wound drainage necessitating irrigation and débridement in two cases, two dislocations, and one refracture. Wong and Gross[40] described the technique and results of 19 patients undergoing an APC reconstruction after a Vancouver type B3 periprosthetic femur fracture. Fifteen patients were available at 5-year follow-up; 13 returned to their preoperative level of function. There was one case of aseptic loosening of the femoral stem and one nonunion of the APC host bone site.

Type C Fracture

Vancouver type C involves fractures occurring well below the tip of the stem. The treatment of choice for these injuries is open reduction and internal fixation of the fracture. Typically, the fracture may be treated independently of the adjacent THA. Locked femoral plating, standard femoral plates, cable plates, retrograde intramedullary nails, and allograft strut plating can be used in treating these fractures. To avoid a stress riser in these cases, we generally recommend that the implant used for fixation overlaps the distal end of the femoral implant, so as not to leave any areas of the femur unprotected.[3] Most published case series include data on type C fractures, with overall good results and fewer complications compared to B1 fractures.[3,41-43]

STRATEGIES TO MINIMIZE COMMON COMPLICATIONS

Periprosthetic fractures of the femur are difficult problems and are increasing in prevalence. Prior surgical procedures often compromise bone quality and the potential for healing, making these fractures difficult to treat. Radiographs typically underestimate the bone loss associated with periprosthetic fractures of the femur and require careful scrutiny.

Prevention of periprosthetic fractures of the femur is critical, and appropriate patient and physician education may go a long way in helping to decrease the number of these fractures in the future. Better treatment and surveillance of osteoporosis may identify and treat those at risk for these pathologic fractures associated with femoral implants with a higher modulus of elasticity. Counseling patients about high-risk activities, particularly younger, more active patients, may help as well. Similarly, intraoperative technique and early recognition of canal penetration, eccentric reaming, and subtle proximal cracks may assist the surgeon in preventing the early periprosthetic fractures.

The causes of late periprosthetic fracture are quite different from the causes of early fracture, as are the means for their prevention. Late fractures typically occur secondary to loose femoral components, osteolysis, osteoporosis, and stress shielding. Most often these fractures are the result of minimal trauma, with

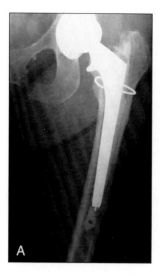
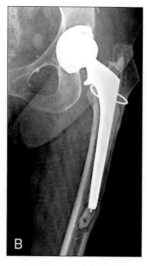

Figure 9 Radiographs of a patient with implant loosening. **A,** AP radiograph of the pelvis shows loosening of the left cemented femoral component, with implant subsidence and cement mantle fracture distally. The patient reported left thigh and knee pain at the time. The primary care physician and radiologist read the radiographs as normal, and the patient was treated with NSAIDs and physical therapy. **B,** One year later, the patient had increasing pain, and this repeat radiograph was obtained, which demonstrates significant varus remodeling and thinning of the lateral femoral cortex.

one of the aforementioned risk factors present. Prevention of these fractures begins with appropriate patient follow-up and surveillance radiographs. In the context of the current US healthcare system, it has been suggested that arthroplasty patients follow up with their primary care physician for routine clinical and radiographic examinations to provide some cost savings to the system. Haddad and associates[44] disagreed with this idea in a recent article, recommending instead that patients continue seeing the surgeon for all follow-up, because the surgeon is better trained to detect silent osteolysis and subtle findings of implant loosening, thereby preventing bone loss/remodeling due to gradual aseptic loosening (**Figure 9**).

Surveillance radiographs should be monitored for eccentric wear of polyethylene components, cement mantle fractures, shedding of the metallic coating, implant subsidence, areas of osteolysis, and osteoporosis. When there is evidence of any of these issues, revision surgery and/or closer surveillance is necessary. We recommend follow-up every 2 years during the first 10 years after surgery and then annually or possibly twice a year thereafter, depending on the radiographic findings and changes from prior radiographs. It is important to have a series of radiographs, including immediate postoperative radiographs, to identify what appears to be a subtle finding. Close surveillance and patient education may help lower the rate of periprosthetic fractures of the femur and decrease the burden this complication of THA places on patients, surgeons, and the healthcare system.

REFERENCES

1. Lewallen DG, Berry DJ: Periprosthetic fracture of the femur after total hip arthroplasty: Treatment and results to date. *Instr Course Lect* 1998;47: 243-249.

2. Berry DJ: Epidemiology: Hip and knee. *Orthop Clin North Am* 1999;30:183-190.

3. Lee SR, Bostrom MP: Periprosthetic fractures of the femur after total hip arthroplasty. *Instr Course Lect* 2004;53:111-118.

4. Schwartz JT, Mayer JG, Engh CA: Femoral fracture during noncemented total hip arthroplasty. *J Bone Joint Surg Am* 1989; 71:1135-1142.

5. Scott RD, Turner RH, Leitzes SM, Aufranc OE: Femoral fractures in conjunction with total hip replacement. *J Bone Joint Surg Am* 1975; 57:494-501.

6. Park MS, Lee YK, Yang KH, Shin SJ: Management of periprosthetic femoral fractures. *J Arthroplasty* 2003;18:903-906.

7. Lindahl H: Epidemiology of periprosthetic femur fracture around a total hip arthroplasty. *Injury* 2007;38:651-654.

8. Berend KR, Lombardi AVJ, Mallory TH, Chonko DJ, Dodds KL, Adams JB: Cerclage wires or cables for the management of intraoperative fracture associated with a cementless, tapered femoral prosthesis: Results at 2 to 16 years. *J Arthroplasty* 2004;19(suppl 2):17-21.

9. Berend ME, Bertrand T: Intra-operative fractures: Rising problems. *Orthopedics* 2007; 30:750-751.

10. Mendenhall S: Hospital resources and implant cost management: A 2004 update. *Orthop Network News* 2004;16.

11. Garbuz DS, Masri BA, Duncan CP: Periprosthetic fractures of the femur: Principles of prevention and management. *Instr Course Lect* 1998;47:237-242.

12. Archibeck MJ, White RE Jr: Learning curve for the two-incision total hip replacement. *Clin Orthop Relat Res* 2004; 429:232-238.

13. Bal BS, Haltom D, Aleto T, Barrett M: Early complications of primary total hip replacement performed with a two-incision minimally invasive technique. *J Bone Joint Surg Am* 2005;87: 2432-2438.

14. Pagnano MW, Leone J, Lewallen DG, Hanssen AD: Two-incision THA had modest outcomes and some substantial complications. *Clin Orthop Relat Res* 2005; 441:86-90.

15. Greidanus NV, Mitchell PA, Masri BA, Garbuz DS, Duncan CP: Principles of management and results of treating the fractured femur during and after total hip arthroplasty. *Instr Course Lect* 2003;52:309-322.

16. Kelley SS: Periprosthetic femoral fractures. *J Am Acad Orthop Surg* 1994;2:164-172.

17. Johansson JE, McBroom R, Barrington TW, Hunter GA: Fracture of the ipsilateral femur in patients with total hip replacement. *J Bone Joint Surg Am* 1981;63:1435-1442.

18. Tsiridis E, Haddad FS, Gie GA: The management of periprosthetic femoral fractures around hip replacements. *Injury* 2003;34: 95-105.

19. Fitzgerald RH Jr, Brindley GW, Kavanagh BF: The uncemented total hip arthroplasty: Intra-operative femoral fractures. *Clin Orthop Relat Res* 1988; 235:61-66.

20. Macdonald SJ, Paprosky WG, Jablonsky WS, Magnus RG: Periprosthetic femoral fractures treated with a long-stem cementless component. *J Arthroplasty* 2001;16:379-383.

21. Beals RK, Tower SS: Periprosthetic fractures of the femur: An analysis of 93 fractures. *Clin Orthop Relat Res* 1996;327:238-246.

22. Larson JE, Chao EY, Fitzgerald RH: Bypassing femoral cortical defects with cemented intramedullary stems. *J Orthop Res* 1991;9:414-421.

23. Moran MC: Treatment of periprosthetic fractures around total hip arthroplasty with an extensively coated femoral component. *J Arthroplasty* 1996;11:981-988.

24. O'Shea K, Quinlan JF, Kutty S, Mulcahy D, Brady OH: The use of uncemented extensively porous-coated femoral components in the management of Vancouver B2 and B3 periprosthetic femoral fractures. *J Bone Joint Surg Br* 2005;87:1617-1621.

25. Springer BD, Berry DJ, Lewallen DG: Treatment of periprosthetic femoral fractures following total hip arthroplasty with femoral component revision. *J Bone Joint Surg Am* 2003;85:2156-2162.

26. Bhattacharyya T, Chang D, Meigs JB, Estok DM II, Malchau H: Mortality after periprosthetic fracture of the femur. *J Bone Joint Surg Am* 2007;89:2658-2662.

27. Lindahl H, Oden A, Garellick G, Malchau H: The excess mortality due to periprosthetic femur fracture: A study from the Swedish national hip arthroplasty register. *Bone* 2007;40:1294-1298.

28. Duncan CP, Masri BA: Fractures of the femur after hip replacement. *Instr Course Lect* 1995;44:293-304.

29. Wang JW, Chen LK, Chen CE: Surgical treatment of fractures of the greater trochanter associated with osteolytic lesions: Surgical technique. *J Bone Joint Surg Am* 2006;88(Suppl 1 Pt 2):250-258.

30. Dennis MG, Simon JA, Kummer FJ, Koval KJ, DiCesare PE: Fixation of periprosthetic femoral shaft fractures occurring at the tip of the stem: A biomechanical study of 5 techniques. *J Arthroplasty* 2000;15:523-528.

31. Haddad FS, Duncan CP, Berry DJ, Lewallen DG, Gross AE, Chandler HP: Periprosthetic femoral fractures around well-fixed implants: Use of cortical onlay allografts with or without a plate. *J Bone Joint Surg Am* 2002;84:945-950.

32. Old AB, McGrory BJ, White RR, Babikian GM: Fixation of Vancouver B1 peri-prosthetic fractures by broad metal plates without the application of strut allografts. *J Bone Joint Surg Br* 2006;88:1425-1429.

33. Buttaro MA, Farfalli G, Paredes Nunez M, Comba F, Piccaluga F: Locking compression plate fixation of Vancouver type-B1 periprosthetic femoral fractures. *J Bone Joint Surg Am* 2007;89: 1964-1969.

34. Sledge JB III, Abiri A: An algorithm for the treatment of Vancouver type B2 periprosthetic proximal femoral fractures. *J Arthroplasty* 2002;17:887-892.

35. Della Valle CJ, Paprosky WG: Classification and an algorithmic approach to the reconstruction of femoral deficiency in revision total hip arthroplasty. *J Bone Joint Surg Am* 2003;85(Suppl 4):1-6.

36. Mulay S, Hassan T, Birtwistle S, Power R: Management of types B2 and B3 femoral periprosthetic fractures by a tapered, fluted, and distally fixed stem. *J Arthroplasty* 2005;20:751-756.

37. Ko PS, Lam JJ, Tio MK, Lee OB, Ip FK: Distal fixation with Wagner revision stem in treating Vancouver type B2 periprosthetic femur fractures in geriatric patients. *J Arthroplasty* 2003;18:446-452.

38. Berry DJ: Treatment of Vancouver B3 periprosthetic femur fractures with a fluted tapered stem. *Clin Orthop Relat Res* 2003;417:224-231.

39. Klein GR, Parvizi J, Rapuri V, et al: Proximal femoral replacement for the treatment of periprosthetic fractures. *J Bone Joint Surg Am* 2005;87:1777-1781.

40. Wong P, Gross AE: The use of structural allografts for treating periprosthetic fractures about the hip and knee. *Orthop Clin North Am* 1999;30:259-264.

41. Sandhu R, Avramidis K, Johnson-Nurse C: Dall-Miles cable and plate fixation system in the treatment of periprosthetic femoral fractures: A review of 20 cases. *J Orthop Surg* (Hong Kong) 2005;13:259-266.

42. Tsiridis E: Dall-Miles plates for periprosthetic femoral fractures: A critical review of 16 cases. *Injury* 2004;35:440-441.

43. Schmidt AH, Kyle RF: Periprosthetic fractures of the femur. *Orthop Clin North Am* 2002;33:143-152.

44. Haddad FS, Ashby E, Konangamparambath S: Should follow-up of patients with arthroplasties be carried out by general practitioners? *J Bone Joint Surg Br* 2007;89:1133-1134.

Chapter 4

LIMB-LENGTH DISCREPANCY

Brian A. Klatt, MD
*Javad Parvizi, MD

CASE PRESENTATION

History

A 58-year-old woman presented with severe pain in the left thigh radiating toward the knee that had started soon after a total hip arthroplasty (THA) performed 6 months earlier. The patient also had sustained two dislocations of the hip—one immediately after surgery while in the recovery room, and the second 2 months later when she rose from a chair. Before presentation to the operating surgeon, the patient had undergone closed reduction and bracing for 6 weeks following each of the two dislocations. A shoe lift had been provided, along with abductor strengthening exercises, as initial management of the limb-length discrepancy (LLD). The patient also had been prescribed analgesics.

The neuralgic pain secondary to the LLD was not responsive to nonsurgical measures, and attempts to ameliorate the LLD with a shoe lift and abductor strengthening had been similarly unsuccessful. An erythrocyte sedimentation rate and C-reactive protein level were obtained; both were normal.

Current Problem

On presentation, clinical examination revealed a true LLD of 3 cm. Plain radiographs showed a cementless total hip implant with a long-neck femoral component in place, with the center of rotation several centimeters above the greater trochanter (**Figure 1**).

DISCUSSION

Recognizing the Problem and High-Risk Situations

LLD following THA can be a significant problem for patients. Although most small LLDs are asymptomatic, some patients with substantial LLDs may expe-

*Javad Parvizi, MD, or the department with which he is affiliated has received research or institutional support from Stryker.

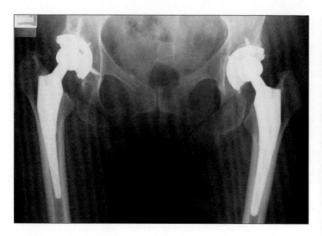

Figure 1 AP pelvic radiograph of a 58-year-old woman with a 3- to 4-cm LLD. Note that the acetabular component in the left hip is positioned more inferiorly and the center of rotation lies above the greater trochanter.

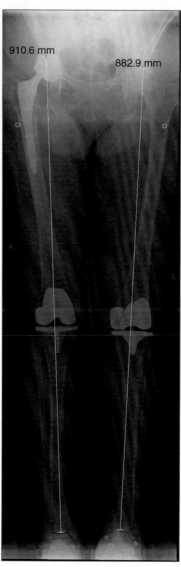

Figure 2 Full-length scanogram used to evaluate true leg length.

rience low back pain or neurogenic pain, sustain a nerve palsy, or have a gait disturbance.[1] Dissatisfaction with leg length is one of the most common reasons for litigation against the orthopaedic community.[2,3]

No precise definition of LLD is agreed upon, and therefore the prevalence of LLD following THA remains unknown. Furthermore, this is an outcome that is dependent on preoperative deformity, surgical technique, and surgical skill. Prevalence rates, therefore, will be a direct result of the surgeon who reports the series. The general consensus is that an LLD >2 cm can be clinically important. One study reported LLD in 14 (16%) of 85 hip replacements.[4] In another study, an average "overlengthening" of >15.9 mm (SD, 9.54 mm) occurred in 144 of 150 hips (96%).[5]

Most clinically symptomatic LLDs following THA are observed during the early postoperative period; often, they resolve with time.[1] In some patients, however, symptomatic LLD persists and is a major contributor to patient dissatisfaction. Patients reporting both true and functional LLD have been studied.[4,6,7] Functional LLD is described as a perception of LLD or feeling of extremity unevenness that occurs despite anatomic equality.[6] Functional LLD is assessed by measuring from the umbilicus to the medial malleolus

of each leg. Functional LLD is often a result of an abduction, adduction, or flexion contracture of the hip or spinal deformity.[8,9] True LLD, on the other hand, results from an anatomic difference in the length of the legs and is often observed as a tilted pelvis or "flexed knee."[8,9] True leg length is measured from the anterior superior iliac spine to the distal aspect of the ipsilateral medial malleolus. If the landmarks are not clear because of soft tissues, a full-length scanogram can be used to evaluate the true leg length (**Figure 2**).

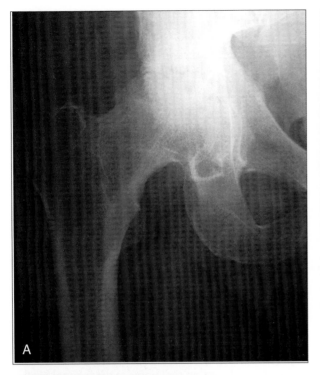

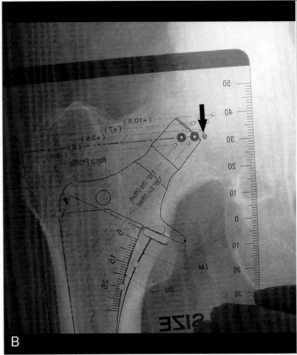

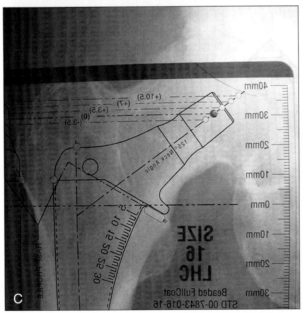

Figure 3 Preoperative assessment of a high-risk patient for LLD. **A,** AP radiograph of a right hip with a varus deformity of the proximal femur, a low neck-shaft angle, and large native femoral offset. **B,** A clear overlay template is used; the desired center of rotation of the hip is marked in pencil (arrow). It is clear that using a standard implant, even with an extended or high-offset option, will not properly restore offset and would risk intraoperative leg lengthening to obtain stability. **C,** A clear overlay template for a "low head center" stem with a lower neck-shaft angle is used; it shows that femoral offset will be properly restored.

Achieving limb-length equality is one of the major objectives of every surgeon performing THA, but postoperative LLD cannot always be avoided. It is important to recognize these situations and to notify the patients of this preoperatively. This includes situations such as preexistent severe limb-length inequality that may occur with developmental dysplasia of the hip or posttraumatic arthritis. There may also be

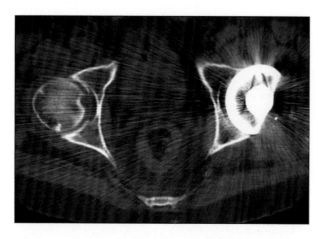

Figure 4 CT scan of the same patient in Figure 1 comfirms the suspected retroversion of the acetabular component.

cases in which hip stability cannot be achieved intraoperatively (despite appropriate component version) without lengthening the leg. Some patients (typically males) have proximal femoral varus, a low neck-shaft angle, and high femoral offset; in these situations, specialized implants may be required to obtain stability and restore offset without substantial lengthening of the leg (**Figure 3**).

Managing Limb-Length Discrepancy

When a patient presents with LLD after a THA, treatment should begin with nonsurgical measures. Functional LLD is a common finding; often this will resolve within the first 6 months. Lumbosacral scoliosis, pelvic obliquity, periarticular muscular spasm, and residual contracture of the hip are examples of functional LLD that may improve with time. Ranawat and Rodriguez[6] drew attention to the concept of functional LLD in a study that showed that despite a high initial incidence, functional LLD persisted in only 1 of 300 replacements done at their institution. They identified only nine patients with persistent functional LLD in 15 years.[6] Patients with a preoperative discrepancy may have contractures that will relax with time, and the body may compensate for many discrepancies without any intervention in the first 6 months. If shoe lifts are used, they should compensate for only the true LLD, to allow the functional LLD to resolve. Physical therapy

with stretching and manipulation has been used to treat functional LLD.

Shoe lifts are another nonsurgical option. For LLD of up to 3/8", a lift placed inside the shoe can be used. For a larger lift, alterations to the heel on the outside of the shoe must be made.

When symptoms do not resolve with nonsurgical measures, revision surgery can be considered. Although revision THA is usually considered as a last resort, recurrent instability, profound functional impairment (secondary to abductor weakness, dysfunctional gait, or low back pain), and failure of nonsurgical treatment may necessitate further surgical intervention. Only patients in whom a problem with component positioning has been identified should be considered candidates for surgical revision.

True LLD is usually a result of component malposition, which either directly or indirectly lengthens the limb.[6] In the case of direct lengthening, the component is placed such that it directly lengthens the limb—for example, an acetabular component that is placed inferior to the anatomic position, or a femoral component that is placed such that the center of the femoral head is substantially proximal to the level of the greater trochanter.

With indirect lengthening, the position of the components in surgery may result in the need to lengthen the limb to achieve stability. For instance, the cup may be placed in retroversion, and the surgeon will compensate for this to achieve stability by placing the femoral component in a proud position or by using a longer femoral ball. Similarly, in the patient with a native hip that has high offset, not restoring offset can lead to leg lengthening to obtain stability. An evaluation of the preoperative radiographs and/or the contralateral native hip will give clues as to the appropriateness of the position of the femoral component by comparing the relative positions of the tip of the greater trochanter and the center of rotation of the hip on the normal and lengthened sides. Further, CT to determine acetabular and femoral component version is useful for identifying component retroversion that could be the etiology of the problem. When such retroversion is identified, it strengthens the case for surgical management (**Figure 4**).

Surgery should address the positioning of the components, and component version is confirmed intraoperatively. Stability will often be improved after version abnormalities are corrected, even with a

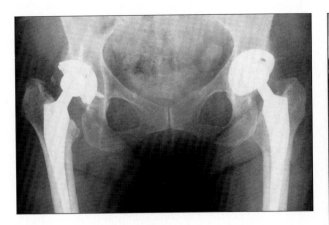

Figure 5 Postoperative radiograph of the patient in Figure 1 after revision to correct the retroversion and inferior positioning of the acetabular component that had led to the underlying LLD. After the surgery, the patient had equal leg lengths.

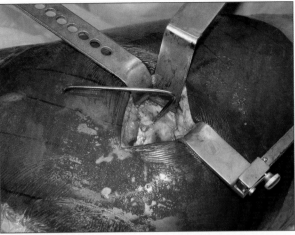

Figure 6 A pin placed in the pelvis is used as a fixed reference point for determining change in leg length during THA.

decrease in length. If stability remains an issue, then the femur can be revised to a higher offset component, or a larger diameter femoral head can be used to augment stability.

A vital component of the preoperative consent process is discussion of LLD issues that may follow THA. The patient should be informed that equal leg length, although desirable, is not always possible. This is especially critical when the patient is at high risk for postoperative LLD, including patients with preoperative deformity or a leg that is longer than the contralateral side preoperatively, or in cases of soft-tissue scarring and chronic limb shortening.

CASE MANAGEMENT
Initial Treatment

A review of the plain radiographs raised the question of retroversion of the acetabular component. The acetabular component also was positioned inferior to the teardrop. CT scans confirmed retroversion of the acetabular component (**Figure 4**). The malpositioned acetabular component was deemed to be the cause of the instability and LLD. It was hypothesized that the malpositioned acetabular component led to intraoperative instability, so the surgeon decided to use a long-neck femoral component to obtain adequate

stability. The left thigh pain was thought to be caused by the lengthening of the limb, which resulted in neuralgic pain in the distribution of the femoral nerve. As the patient had experienced recurrent instability, persistent neuralgic pain, and a large symptomatic LLD, revision surgery was elected as the most appropriate course of treatment.

At the time of revision surgery, retroversion of the acetabular component was confirmed. The cup was removed and repositioned in the appropriate anteversion. At the conclusion of the surgery, leg lengths were restored to equal.

Outcome/Follow-up

With proper alignment of the cup (**Figure 5**), stability was improved and the patient did not experience any further dislocations. The anterior thigh pain resolved by the first follow-up appointment.

STRATEGIES TO MINIMIZE COMMON COMPLICATIONS

To avoid LLD after THA, proper preoperative planning and appropriate execution of the procedure are essential. The acetabular and femoral components should be placed in the desired positions, and hip stability and equal limb length should be confirmed intraoperatively. Preoperatively, a physical examination and plain radiographs will provide the information needed to equalize leg lengths. The standard AP pelvis view will reveal significant collapse, dislocation, or shortening that would challenge the possibility of restoring leg length. Offset of the hip also can be assessed on plain radiographs, and restoration of proper offset aids in avoiding LLD. An appropriate amount of femoral offset will restore tension to the soft tissues and abductors. If this tension is not restored, it will lead to the necessity of intraoperative lengthening to attain hip stability.

Leg length is in large part determined by the placement of the components. If the hip center of rotation is accurately restored and the acetabular component is placed in the "anatomic" position, equal leg length should result. The recommended anteversion for placement of the femoral component is 10° to 15°; for the acetabular component, it is 15° to 25°.[10] The inclination of the cup should be between 35° and 50°.[10] Deviations from these recommendations and individualization may at times be necessary, however, to reproduce the "anatomy" of the patient. By identifying the acetabular and femoral anatomy during surgery, the location of the cup and stem can be reliably placed in the proper position. Using this anatomic information, the version can be restored correctly and a stable hip obtained. When intraoper-ative instability is noted, the position of the components should be scrutinized before resorting to neck lengthening and tensioning of the soft tissues.

Leg length should be assessed following insertion of the trial component and, of course, at the conclusion of surgery. Performing THA with the patient in the supine position may allow for better assessment of the leg length by direct palpation of the anterior superior iliac spine and the medial malleoli. Surgeons who place the patient in the lateral position often use indirect measures to assess leg length in addition to using preoperative templating to determine the placement of the acetabular component and the height of the femoral neck osteotomy. Many techniques have been used to intraoperatively assess leg lengths; most involve placing a pin or other fixed point in the pelvis (usually the ilium) and using it to reference the relative position of a marked point on the femur before surgical dislocation and following placement of the trial components (**Figure 6**). This technique measures the change in leg length, but it does not directly compare the length of the leg to the contralateral side. More recently, computer-guided navigation systems have been introduced that reportedly allow for better assessment of component position and also leg length. It is possible that the use of such navigation may help to avoid LLD following THA.

REFERENCES

1. Parvizi J, Sharkey PF, Bissett GA, Rothman RH, Hozack WJ: Surgical treatment of limb-length discrepancy following total hip arthroplasty. *J Bone Joint Surg Am* 2003;85-A:2310-2317.

2. Clark CR, Huddleston HD, Schoch EP III, Thomas BJ: Leg-length discrepancy after total hip arthroplasty. *J Am Acad Orthop Surg* 2006;14:38-45.

3. Hofmann AA, Skrzynski MC: Leg-length inequality and nerve palsy in total hip arthroplasty: A lawyer awaits! *Orthopedics* 2000;23:943-944.

4. Jasty M, Webster W, Harris W: Management of limb length inequality during total hip replacement. *Clin Orthop Relat Res* 1996;333:165-171.

5. Williamson JA, Reckling FW: Limb length discrepancy and related problems following total hip joint replacement. *Clin Orthop Relat Res* 1978;134: 135-138.

6. Ranawat CS, Rodriguez JA: Functional leg-length inequality following total hip arthroplasty. *J Arthroplasty* 1997;12:359-364.

7. Edeen J, Sharkey PF, Alexander AH: Clinical significance of leg-length inequality after total hip arthroplasty. *Am J Orthop* 1995;24:347-351.

8. Knutson GA: Anatomic and functional leg-length inequality: A review and recommendation for clinical decision-making. Part I: anatomic leg-length inequality. Prevalence, magnitude, effects and clinical significance. *Chiropr Osteopat* 2005;13:11.

9. Knutson GA: Anatomic and functional leg-length inequality: A review and recommendation for clinical decision-making. Part II: the functional or unloaded leg-length asymmetry. *Chiropr Osteopat* 2005;13:12.

10. Lewinnek GE, Lewis JL, Tarr R, et al: Dislocations after total hip-replacement arthroplasties. *J Bone Joint Surg Am* 1978;60: 217-220.

INSTABILITY

Todd Sekundiak, MD, FRCSC

The goals of total hip arthroplasty (THA) include the re-creation of normal hip biomechanics to minimize joint reactive forces while improving motor function, in an effort to optimize the likelihood of long-term durability of the construct. When THA fails to reproduce a normal anatomic hip, secondary to the surgical technique used or the choice of implant, prosthetic dislocation can occur.

CASE PRESENTATION

History

A 50-year-old female smoker weighing 110 lb (50 kg) presented with a painful, degenerative kyphoscoliosis, a seronegative arthropathy of unknown origin, and polyarticular joint disease; she was a household ambulator. To control the back pain, a spinal fusion was attempted that unfortunately resulted in a pseudarthrosis and further back pain, with a resultant kyphotic deformity of 80°. The chronic back pain had led to chronic and progressive narcotic use and eventual dependency.

Subsequently, the patient's left hip became symptomatic and a THA was performed. The hip dislocated initially 3 months postoperatively, and the dislocations became recurrent. The provocative mechanism was unclear, but these dislocations commonly occurred while the patient was sitting. In this patient, initial attempts at bracing had been unsuccessful because of skin breakdown and noncompliance. Radiographs showed that both index components were cementless, modular, and bone-ingrown. The original operating surgeon returned the patient to the operating room and performed an acetabular revision with exchange of the modular femoral head. Unfortunately, the hip continued to dislocate posteriorly, and a second opinion was sought (**Figure 1**).

Presentation of the Complication

The patient presented to my institution in a wheelchair. On physical examination, she was oriented but presented with slurred speech and seemed somnolent secondary to narcotic use. Eye contact was difficult because of the severe fixed kyphotic deformity. Her extremities were neurovascularly intact and the

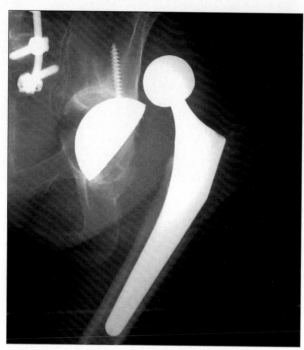

Figure 1 AP radiograph of the left hip of the patient described in the case presentation demonstrates dislocation after revision THA.

prior skin incision was well healed, without signs of infection. Her muscle mass was so poor that the femoral head could be palpated in the left buttock region. The patient was unable to stand, and the extremity was measured clinically as approximately 3 cm shorter than the contralateral extremity. Range of motion of the hip produced significant pain. Girdlestone resection arthroplasty and further non-surgical treatment were discussed with the patient; however, she desired revision surgery. An erythrocyte sedimentation rate and C-reactive protein level were obtained; both were negative for infection.

DISCUSSION
Recognizing the Problem and High-Risk Situation

Although rates of dislocation after THA have decreased with improvements in surgical technique, implant design, and bearing surface technologies that allow for larger femoral heads, dislocation continues to be one of the most common complications following THA, with rates ranging from 0.2% to 7% after primary THA.[1,2] Revision THA fares even worse, with reported rates of instability up to 25% in some series.[3] It has been estimated that closed reduction of a dislocated hip adds 19% to the cost of the index procedure, and an open reduction is likely to add 150%. Most dislocations present early (within 3 months); however, the initial dislocation can occur many years after the index procedure. von Knoch and associates[4] reported that up to 32% of initial dislocations occurred 5 or more years after the index procedure. These late dislocations were associated with a history of symptoms of subluxation, a traumatic episode, cognitive impairment, wear of the bearing surface, component loosening, and component malposition. Fifty-five percent of these dislocations became recurrent.[4]

Patient-Related Factors

Because of limitations inherent to most traditional implants, patients are routinely instructed to follow "hip precautions" postoperatively. Until the pericapsular soft tissues are healed and a strong soft-tissue envelope is developed, patients are at an increased risk of dislocation during this early rehabilitative phase. Cognitive inability to follow hip precautions, both early and late, is believed to increase the risk of dislocation.

Cognitive impairment can take many forms, including drug dependencies and alcoholism. Patients with a history of alcohol abuse have been shown to have a fivefold increased risk of dislocation. Neuromuscular disorders, such as Parkinson's disease, epilepsy, cerebral palsy, and muscular dystrophy, can produce involuntary motions of the hip and place the patient at risk of dislocation. Advanced age may lead to an increased risk of falls, decreased muscle control, and degradation of cognitive abilities, all of which can increase the risk of dislocation. The notion that age in and of itself is related causally to dislocation is controversial, however. Some authors believe that obesity, gender, age, height, and preoperative diagnosis are not risk factors for dislocation; however, Lübbeke and associates[5] found a 2.4-fold increased relative risk of dislocation in obese women compared to their nonobese counterparts. Similarly, in another study, a diagnosis of inflammatory arthropathies increased the odds ratio of a dislocation to 3.7 compared with a preoperative diagnosis of degenerative arthritis.[6]

Implants

Femoral head size has long been discussed as a factor relating to hip dislocation, but clinical studies have not supported this relationship.[2] These initial comparisons were made between traditional head sizes of 26, 28, and 32 mm. There is presently a better understanding of relative head-neck ratios and head-cup ratios that mechanically determine the arc of hip motion that can occur before the femoral and acetabular component will impinge, lever, and ultimately dislocate. Laboratory studies have shown improved range of motion when head size increases from 22 to 28 mm.[7] Larger heads were precluded in the past because of concerns about premature wear of traditional polyethylene. With the introduction of cross-linked polyethylene and alternative bearing surfaces, 36-, 38-, 40-, and 44-mm heads could be used. The reported wear rates with these materials and head sizes are promising, and dislocation rates should also be diminished. Peters and associates[8] compared 28-mm and 38-mm heads and found 2.5% versus 0% dislocation rates, respectively, when used in primary THA. With metal-on-metal articulations using femoral heads within 6 to 8 mm of the outer diameter of the acetabular component, dislocation rates of less than 1% have been reported in several series.[8] Larger femoral heads not only increase the distance the femoral head must travel out of the acetabulum before dislocation will occur (the so-called jump distance) but also increase the range of motion before contact between the femoral head and the acetabular component occurs. This improves the jump distance, head-neck ratio, and head–acetabular component ratio.

A better understanding of head-neck ratios also has led to implant modifications. It is not the size of the head in isolation but rather how the head and neck relate to the acetabulum that influences the risk of dislocation.[9] Skirted femoral heads are routinely avoided because of the concern that the skirt will impinge on the rim of the acetabulum and lever the head out of the acetabulum. A skirt has been shown to decrease the arc of hip motion by 10° to 15° in all planes compared to an unskirted head.[10] For the same size head, this arc of motion is also diminished when the cup becomes larger. This can translate to increased dislocation rates when smaller femoral heads are used with larger acetabular components. Hence, given the improved wear performance of modern bearing surfaces, many surgeons now recommend the use of larger-diameter femoral heads in larger cups to improve the arc of motion before the neck impinges on the rim of the cup.[9] Manufacturers have even modified the femoral necks (making them trapezoidal rather than circular) in hopes of improving range of motion without diminishing structural integrity.

Elevated-rim acetabular liners have been shown to decrease the risk of dislocation.[11] An elevated rim, however, does decrease the arc of motion in the direction opposite from where the rim is placed and thus can cause instability in the opposite direction (eg, an elevated rim posteriorly can increase the risk of anterior dislocation). Further, impingement of the prosthetic femoral neck against an elevated rim can cause substantial nonarticular surface wear, which is a concern with these implants as well.

To avoid these suboptimal constructs, increased offset options are offered on both the acetabular and femoral side. These components can be used to increase tension in the soft-tissue sleeve without compromising leg length.[1] Any hip can be made stable; the important point is that it must be made stable without increasing leg length or femoral offset beyond the patient's normal anatomy. Increasing length or offset beyond what is normal will not only create cosmetic (and potential legal) problems but may also produce pain secondary to placing undue tension on the soft tissues.

Surgical Technique

Posterior approaches to the hip have been reported to have a higher dislocation rate (1% to 9.5%) than the lateral and anterolateral approaches (0% to 3.3%).[1-4,12] Newer techniques have a reported dislocation rate of 0% to 2% with the posterior approach.[12] This improvement in dislocation rates has been attributed to a change in surgical technique: capsulotomy and associated capsular repair are being peformed rather than a complete or partial capsulectomy.[12] This suggests that surgical technique may

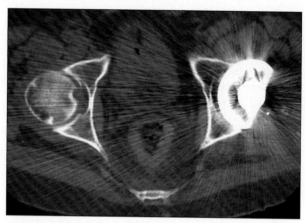

Figure 2   CT scan demonstrates a retroverted acetabular component.

play a larger role than the approach itself. Similarly, Shervin and associates[13] reviewed 26 articles on outcomes after THA and concluded that both surgeon volume and hospital volume were associated with postoperative dislocation rates, with the surgeon volume weighing more heavily.

Component positioning is one of the most critical issues in determining hip stability and one of the most difficult to reproduce. Authors have advocated 15° ± 10° of anteversion and 40° ± 10° of lateral flexion to promote stability.[14] Unfortunately, this range of stable positions does not imply inherent hip stability. Both femoral and acetabular component malposition can alter stability.[1,2,14]

Integrity of both the static and dynamic stabilizers of the hip is critical to maintaining hip stability. The importance of the capsular structures has already been discussed. Similarly, the integrity of the hip abductors is critical to maintaining hip stability. Disruption of the abductor mass can occur with difficult or minimally invasive approaches. Most commonly, disruption of the greater trochanter occurs, causing functional disruption of the abductors and an increased risk of dislocation.

Management of the Unstable THA
Initial Evaluation

Initial evaluation should include a thorough history and physical examination to confirm the mechanism

and direction of the dislocation. Closed treatment may be indicated in a patient who presents with an initial dislocation and in whom considerable force is required to reproduce symptoms; surgical treatment is more likely to be appropriate in patients with recurrent dislocations and in whom symptoms are elicited with minimal effort. The mechanism of the dislocation will help determine the direction of the dislocation and methodology for the relocation. Knowing the mechanism also helps in interpreting the radiographs to determine component position and bone or soft-tissue abnormalities. Rarely are further investigations required. If the patient can tolerate the procedure, a shoot-through lateral radiograph will confirm the direction of the dislocation. CT can be used to specifically determine both femoral and acetabular component orientation and help plan the revision procedure for repositioning of the components (**Figure 2**). Documentation of neurovascular status of the extremity and the status of the implants is critical before performing reduction maneuvers.

Nonsurgical Treatment

An initial early postsurgical dislocation can usually be treated with closed reduction as long as the femoral and acetabular components are well positioned and not loose, although the surgeon should realize and inform the patient that there is an increased risk of redislocation, with a recurrence rate of up to 38%.[1-4] For closed reduction to be successful, it is important to provide adequate muscular relaxation as well as analgesia. Numerous "cocktails" have been suggested, but regardless of the type used, initial traction to the involved extremity should not evoke a voluntary or involuntary contraction of the musculature. It is critical to ensure that the dynamic hip stabilizers are overcome with the reduction maneuver and that no damage occurs to the components or the patient's own tissues with the reduction. Both failed and successful reductions have been shown to cause damage to the components. Both macroscopic and microscopic damage to the bearing surface could lead to further instability or compromised long-term viability of the arthroplasty. If adequate relaxation cannot be obtained in the emergency department setting, then the reduction should be performed under anesthesia in the operating room. Again, it is essential that the anesthetist be directed to provide adequate muscular relaxation, not just sedation, to aid in obtaining the reduction.

The technique used for the reduction is dependent on the direction of the dislocation, with reduction usually performed with longitudinal traction in line with the dislocation. Reduction techniques after THA are similar to the maneuvers for traumatic dislocations of the native hip. The rotation associated with the dislocation is initially exaggerated while traction is maintained. For posterior dislocations, the hip tends to be kept in a flexed and adducted position until the cusp of the reduction, when rotation should be corrected to neutral. For an anterior dislocation, the hip is extended (or slightly flexed) and externally rotated. External rotation is maintained until a reduction is obtained with longitudinal traction. Intraoperative fluoroscopy can be used to evaluate the success of the maneuvers and the stability and status of the implants, as well as potential incarceration of implants. Although the use of abduction braces and knee immobilizers following successful reduction has been promoted, their support in the peer-reviewed literature has been scant. If the reduction is successful and no alteration in neurovascular or implant status occurs, then immediate weight bearing can occur. If compromise to the extremity's neurovascular status occurs, emergent exploration is indicated because of possible incarceration. If radiography reveals damage to the implants, urgent exploration is similarly indicated.

Surgical Treatment

Surgical treatment is indicated for recurrent dislocations when components are malpositioned or loose. Recurrence of dislocation and associated soft-tissue or bony abnormalities are additional indications. If the components are well positioned, attempts at removing sources of soft-tissue or bony impingement, along with modular component exchange, can be successful in most cases. With most components being modular, other options can be used to promote stability while one or both components are repositioned. Modularity allows for alteration in neck length, acetabular offset, and head diameter. As discussed earlier, elevated rims or femoral head skirts

are not recommended. Increasing femoral head diameter promotes stability by itself, but it also provides increased neck length without early incorporation of a skirt as compared to a smaller-diameter head of equal length. A large head alone can rarely correct recurrent instabilities when other issues exist, however, such as malpositioned components or deficient abductor mechanisms.[15]

The component that is most malpositioned should be revised, although revision of both components may be required. In general, the acetabular component is more likely to be malpositioned than the femoral component. Femoral revision is also less appealing given the relative ease of removing a well-fixed acetabular component with modern instrumentation compared with the morbidity associated with removing a well-fixed femoral component and the resultant bone and soft-tissue destruction that can occur and lead to an increased risk of dislocation. However, if the femoral component is modular, easily revisable, or loose, then it should unquestionably be revised if malpositioned. Isolated liner exchange should be performed with caution, as this may actually lead to increased risk of rerevision and recurrence of dislocations, particularly if femoral head size is not maximized.

Trochanteric nonunion, malunion, or scar can also lead to dislocation by introducing femoral-pelvic impingement before prosthetic neck and acetabular impingement occurs. This will promote early levering of the articulation and resultant dislocation in physiologic ranges of motion. It is important to correct the bony deformities and attempt union of the trochanter to its anatomic base. Even if union fails to occur, a stable fibrous nonunion in an anatomic position is less likely to cause dislocation. If this cannot be achieved, the surgeon is advised to enucleate the displaced trochanter to prevent bony impingement from occurring. Similarly, scar or any other bony excrescence that impedes motion or promotes impingement necessitates removal of the offending tissue.

Multiple ancillary procedures have been advocated to prevent or correct dislocation, but many patients continue to experience instability after undergoing these procedures. For example, with well-positioned implants, trochanteric advancement has been described. This aims to overtension the abductors from their normal anatomic position. This

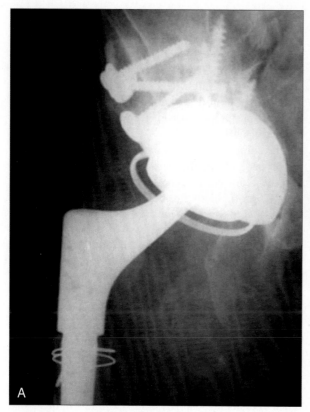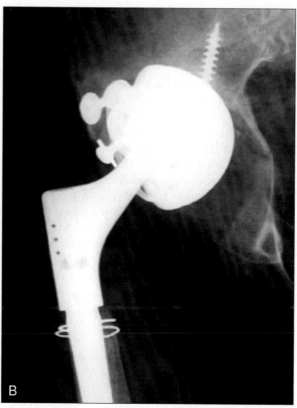

Figure 3 AP radiographs of a right hip after THA using a constrained acetabular liner. **A,** Initial postoperative radiograph. **B,** Postoperative radiograph at 6 weeks, showing catastrophic failure of the acetabular component.

procedure is recommended only in a pathologic hip that cannot be normalized. Routine advancement will likely produce chronic pain because the muscles will be constantly under undue stress. Achilles tendon allograft and bone blocks that act as check reins, to block motion beyond what is felt to be safe for the arthroplasty construct, also have been described in small, single-surgeon series.

Constrained acetabular liners continue to gain popularity because of their ease of use, but they are associated with problems of their own. Berend and associates[16] reported on 755 constrained liners and found them effective in preventing recurrent dislocation in 71.1% of patients. Constrained acetabular liners should be considered only in salvage situations, however, because most designs are associated with limited range of motion, which can lead to premature femoral neck and acetabular rim impingement. If this

limitation is small and nonphysiologic for the patient, the liner will be successful, but if the limitation is significant, continual neck-acetabular contact will occur, leading to fatigue failure of the mechanism or, worse yet, catastrophic failure of the acetabular component itself (**Figure 3**). Constrained acetabular components are indicated in recurrent dislocators who have inadequate soft-tissue constraints but no other dislocating factors.

It is important to recognize that not all constrained liners are the same; different rates of success are reported in the literature for different designs. Goetz and associates[17] have reported long-term success with a tripolar constrained component, with only 7% of patients having recurrent dislocations, and an overall complication rate of 21%. If the acetabular component is not made to mechanically lock onto these liners, cementing the liners into the

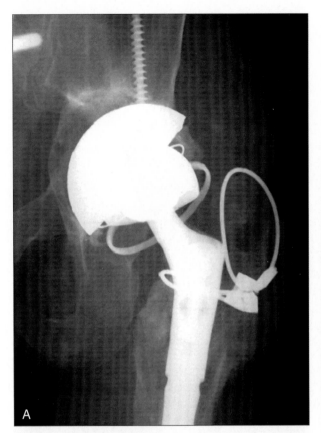 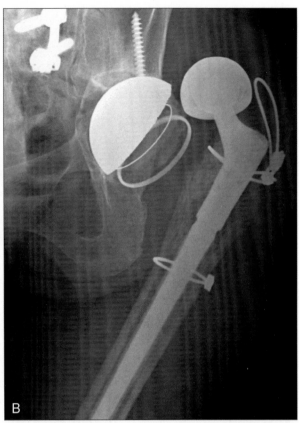

Figure 4 AP radiographs of the patient described in the case presentation after revision of the femoral component and insertion of a constrained liner. **A,** Postoperative radiograph shows the components in place. **B,** Radiograph demonstrates recurrent posterior dislocation following revision.

components can be performed with reasonable success. A well-positioned component should be ensured to prevent impingement.

CASE SUMMARY

Management

When the patient presented, she had undergone revision of the acetabular component, but because of ongoing instability, the repeat revision was performed. The direction of instability was difficult to determine from the history, but clinically it appeared to be posterior. The acetabular component was ingrown and in a neutrally anteverted position. The femoral component was noted to be ingrown and

retroverted. Because of fear of further acetabular bone loss and the known oblique nature of the capture mechanism, the acetabular component was left in situ and the femoral component was revised (**Figure 4,** *A*). Significant compromise to the abductor mechanism occurred with revision of the femoral component, further compromising the stability of the hip.

Outcome

Unfortunately, the patient had recurrent instability with dissociation of the constrained mechanism (**Figure 4,** *B*). Attempts to retain the components and use a different constrained liner (by cementing it into the shell) similarly failed to produce stability (**Fig-**

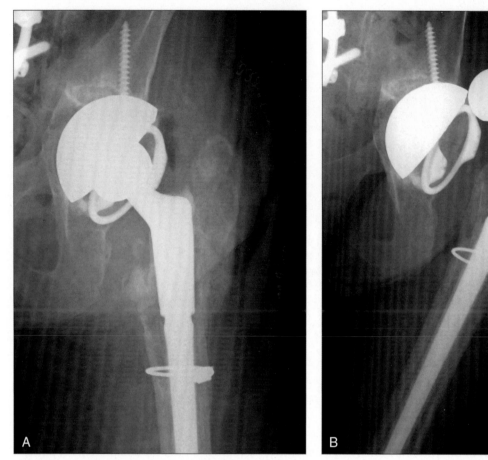

Figure 5 AP radiographs of the patient described in the case presentation after further revision surgery with cementation of a different constrained liner into the well-fixed acetabular metal shell. **A,** Postoperative radiograph shows the components in place. **B,** Radiograph demonstrates recurrent dislocation.

ure 5). The patient history revealed overdosing with narcotics, resulting in a state of altered consciousness that caused the patient to sit with her head between her knees. Modification of narcotic use and reorientation of the acetabular component into appropriate anteversion prevented the anterior impingement and posterior dislocation, and the patient was dislocation-free at 2-year follow-up (**Figure 6**).

SUMMARY

Instability continues to be a dominant complication and cause of failure after THA. Immaculate surgical

technique and appropriate implant selection are necessary to prevent iatrogenic instability. Postoperatively, patients unfortunately must alter their activities to avoid provocative maneuvers that will lead to hip dislocation. When dislocation occurs, the key is to determine its etiology and, if component position is adequate, safely perform a closed reduction without damaging the bearing surface or the surrounding soft tissues. If component malposition or soft-tissue insufficiency is suspected and dislocations recur, surgical correction is indicated. If component reorientation does not correct the instability, or if abductor insufficiency is present, then salvage techniques such as constrained implants are indicated.

As techniques and implants improve, THA patients may begin to lead more normal lifestyles without the fear of instability, but this is not yet reality. In the future, however, with better imaging techniques and improved prosthetic implants, the surgeon may be able to "tailor fit" the implant to the patient's physiologic needs. Creation of a dynamic image of the hip preoperatively will help determine the physical needs of the patient and prevent dislocation or correct its cause. Similarly, a dynamic three-dimensional picture of the hip with the implants positioned will be created preoperatively to ensure that the component type and position are best suited to that patient. It will then be the surgeon's job to match this template with tools such as robotic navigation to ensure the most physiologic hip possible.

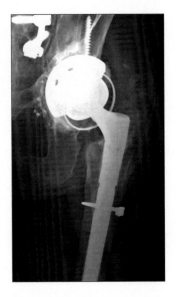

Figure 6 AP radiograph of the patient described in the case presentation 2 years after revision surgery to appropriately antevert the acetabular component.

REFERENCES

1. Soong M, Rubash HE, Macaulay W: Dislocation after total hip arthroplasty. *J Am Acad Orthop Surg* 2004;12:314-321.
2. McCollum DE, Gray WJ: Dislocation after total hip arthroplasty: Causes and prevention. *Clin Orthop Relat Res* 1990;261:159-170.
3. Alberton GM, High WA, Morrey BF: Dislocation after revision total hip arthroplasty: An analysis of risk factors and treatment options. *J Bone Joint Surg Am* 2002;84:1788-1792.
4. von Knoch M, Berry DJ, Harmsen WS, Morrey BF: Late dislocation after total hip arthroplasty. *J Bone Joint Surg Am* 2002;84:1949-1953.
5. Lübbeke A, Stern R, Garavaglia G, Zurcher L, Hoffmeyer P: Differences in outcomes of obese women and men undergoing primary total hip arthroplasty. *Arthritis Rheum* 2007;57:327-334.
6. Zwartele RE, Brand R, Doets HC: Increased risk of dislocation after primary total hip arthroplasty in inflammatory arthritis: A prospective observational study of 410 hips. *Acta Orthop Scand* 2004;75:684-690.
7. Bartz RL, Nobel PC, Kadakia NR, Tullos HS: The effect of femoral component head size on posterior dislocation of the artificial hip joint. *J Bone Joint Surg Am* 2000;82:1300-1307.
8. Peters CL, McPherson E, Jackson JD, Erickson JA: Reduction in early dislocation rate with large-diameter femoral heads in primary total hip arthroplasty. *J Arthroplasty* 2007;22:140-144.
9. Kelley SS, Lachiewicz PF, Hickman JM, Paterno SM: Relationship of femoral head and acetabular size to the prevalence of dislocation. *Clin Orthop Relat Res* 1998;355:163-170.
10. Kluess D, Martin H, Mittelmeier W, Schmitz KP, Bader R: Influence of femoral head size on impingement, dislocation and stress distribution in total hip replacement. *Med Eng Phys* 2007;29:465-471.
11. Cobb TK, Morrey BF, Ilstrup DM: The elevated-rim acetabular liner in total hip arthroplasty: Relationship to postoperative dislocation. *J Bone Joint Surg Am* 1996;78:80-86.
12. Goldstein WM, Gleason TF, Kopplin M, Branson JJ: Prevalence of dislocation after total hip arthroplasty through a posterolateral approach with partial capsulotomy and capsulorrhaphy. *J Bone Joint Surg Am* 2001;83:2-7.
13. Shervin N, Rubash HE, Katz JN: Orthopaedic procedure volume and patient outcomes: A systematic literature review. *Clin Orthop Relat Res* 2007;457:35-41.
14. Biedermann R, Tonin A, Krismer M, Rachbauer F, Eibl G, Stöckl B: Reducing the risk of dislocation

after total hip arthroplasty: The effect of orientation of the acetabular component. *J Bone Joint Surg Br* 2005;87:762-769.

15. Lachiewicz PF, Soileau ES: Dislocation of primary total hip arthroplasty with 36 and 40-mm heads. *Clin Orthop Relat Res* 2006;453:153-155.

16. Berend KR, Lombardi AV, Mallory TH, Adams JB, Russell JH, Groseth KL: The long-term outcome of 755 consecutive constrained acetabular components in total hip arthroplasty: Examining the successes and failures. *J Arthroplasty* 2005;20: 93-102.

17. Goetz DD, Bremner BR, Callaghan JJ, Capello WN, Johnston RC: Salvage of a recurrently dislocating total hip prosthesis with use of a constrained acetabular component: A concise follow-up of a previous report. *J Bone Joint Surg Am* 2004;86: 2419-2423.

Chapter 6

PERIPROSTHETIC INFECTION

Craig J. Della Valle, MD

CASE 1: ACUTE POSTOPERATIVE INFECTION

History

A 57-year-old woman with a history significant for diabetes mellitus and a body mass index of 52 presented with right hip pain that was recalcitrant to nonsurgical treatment. Physical examination and plain radiographs confirmed end-stage arthritis of the right hip. A right total hip arthroplasty (THA) was performed, and the immediate postoperative course was uncomplicated.

The patient presented to the office on postoperative day 17 with new drainage from the distal part of the incision (it had previously been dry) with surrounding erythema. The patient was afebrile but reported an increase in pain in addition to the drainage. Plain radiographs showed no interval change compared to radiographs obtained in the recovery room. Given the patient's history of new drainage and the appearance of the wound, the patient was brought to the fluoroscopy suite for a hip aspiration; 10 mL of fluid was obtained and sent for a synovial fluid white blood cell (WBC) count with differential and aerobic, anaerobic, fungal, and culture for acid-fast bacilli. Other laboratory work included a complete blood count, erythrocyte sedimentation rate (ESR), and C-reactive protein (CRP).

The ESR and CRP were both highly elevated; the peripheral WBC count was normal. The synovial fluid WBC count was 28,000, with 92% polymorphonuclear cells (PMNs). Based on the synovial fluid cell count, the patient was brought urgently to the operating room that evening, where an irrigation and débridement was performed including a modular exchange of the polyethylene liner and femoral head. The wound was closed using absorbable, nonbraided sutures over two drains, one placed deep to and one superficial to the fascia. An infectious disease consult was obtained and empiric vancomycin was started in

*Craig J. Della Valle, MD, or the department with which he is affiliated has received research or institutional support from Zimmer, miscellaneous nonincome support, commercially derived honoraria, or other nonresearch-related funding from Zimmer, Stryker, and Smith & Nephew, and is a consultant for or an employee of Zimmer.

the operating room after the three sets of surgical cultures were obtained. All three sets of surgical cultures grew methicillin-sensitive *Staphylococcus aureus*; antibiotic therapy was changed to cefazolin. The patient was treated with 6 weeks of intravenous antibiotics and then transitioned to oral cephalexin.

The patient presented 9 weeks after the irrigation and débridement with new drainage from the wound and increased pain. Radiographs showed no interval change.

Case Management and Outcome

The hip was reaspirated and the synovial fluid WBC count was 34,500 with 85% PMNs. The patient was subsequently brought back to the operating room, where a resection arthroplasty was performed and an antibiotic-loaded spacer was placed. After the patient completed another 6-week course of intravenous antibiotics, a successful reimplantation was performed.

Discussion

Recognizing the Problem and High-Risk Situations

The primary risk factors for postoperative infection of a THA include obesity, diabetes mellitus, inflammatory arthritis (such as rheumatoid arthritis), chronic renal failure, malnutrition, skin disorders that compromise its integrity (such as psoriasis), steroid dependency, and other disorders that lead to immunocompromise. One study also found the use of low molecular-weight heparin for thromboembolic prophylaxis to be associated with an increased risk of postoperative wound infection following THA.[1]

Diagnosis of Acute Postoperative Infection

Diagnosis of an early postoperative infection following THA can be difficult because the signs may be subtle and diagnostic tests may be difficult to interpret in the early postoperative period. Persistent wound drainage is a common sign; in one study, approximately 20% of hip wounds had some drainage at 5 days

postoperatively.[1] These same authors, however, found wound drainage to be an important harbinger of infection, with each day of wound drainage increasing the risk of wound infection by more than 40%.

In some cases, the diagnosis of infection is obvious because the patient presents with a wound that is draining purulent-appearing fluid, has systemic symptoms (such as fever), and reports a pattern of increasing pain. Conversely, in most patients who have scant amounts of clear drainage that is decreasing in volume, appropriate management comprises discontinuation of anticoagulation therapy, local treatment of the wound with frequent dressing changes and painting with betadine, and careful observation. The indiscriminate use of oral antibiotics is to be avoided because they can mask a deep infection that requires surgical treatment, resulting in a delay of appropriate treatment. Similarly, swabbing of the skin around a draining wound for culture provides little useful information and is discouraged.

When an acute postoperative infection is suspected but cannot be confirmed on clinical grounds, the best test available is an aspiration of the hip joint performed under fluoroscopic guidance. The aspirated fluid is sent for a synovial fluid WBC count with differential and culture (aerobic, anaerobic, fungal, and for acid-fast bacilli). Results from my institution have shown that the synovial fluid WBC count can be particularly useful for identifying an infection.[2] If the cell count is >9,000 and the differential shows >80% PMNs, infection is likely; conversely, WBC counts of <3,000 are usually not associated with infection. If equivocal values are obtained, the surgeon can admit the patient to the hospital and initiate intravenous antibiotic treatment (after the hip has been aspirated), awaiting final culture results to assist in the decision-making process. If fluid cannot be obtained at the time of aspiration, the patient is admitted to the hospital for careful monitoring of temperature and wound drainage. If the wound drainage does not subside, the patient is returned to the operating room for débridement and exploration of the wound.

Managing Acute Postoperative Infection

Superficial wound débridements should be avoided in the setting of early periprosthetic infection because if infection is present, it is rarely, if ever, isolated to the area above the deep fascia. The fascia of the gluteus maximus is thin proximally and difficult to close securely, and thus if the wound is opened in the operating room, the deep fascia should be opened completely. All suture material is removed and three sets of cultures are obtained from around the implants along with another fluid aspiration, often through the deep fascia.

Options at this point include a thorough irrigation and débridement with retention of well-fixed components (including exchange of all modular parts such as the femoral head and liner), a direct (ie, one-stage) component exchange, or removal of the components and placement of an antibiotic-loaded spacer (two-stage exchange). Unfortunately, little information is available to guide the orthopaedic surgeon in the appropriate course of action. The results of irrigation and débridement with component retention in general seem to be poor, particularly if cementless components have been implanted at the time of the index procedure,[3,4] with overall success rates for the procedure approximating 50%. Patients treated with this approach should be clearly informed that further surgery and eventual implant removal might be required. Multiple attempts at débridement should not be attempted; if the wound fails to heal after the initial débridement, the surgeon should proceed with a two-stage exchange. Patients should be given the option of proceeding directly to a two-stage exchange, for which reported rates of infection eradication are generally 90% or better.[4] Little information is available on direct component exchange in this setting; however, the use of antibiotic-loaded cement for component fixation seems to be associated with improved results.[5]

If irrigation and débridement is selected as the treatment of choice, the modular femoral head is carefully removed, taking care to not damage the Morse taper (**Figure 1**); removal of the femoral head improves access for further débridement. A complete synovectomy is performed and tissue is sent for intraoperative frozen section. Unfortunately, no good data are available on what the criteria for infection in the early postoperative period should be; however, the histopathology does present another data point for interpreting the overall picture. If a modular liner is present, this is likewise removed and stability of the components is ensured; loose components must be removed and an

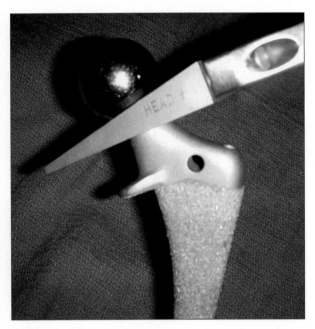

Figure 1   A tool such as the Versys Head/Neck Separator (Zimmer, Warsaw, IN) is used to remove the modular femoral head without damaging the Morse taper.

antibiotic spacer placed. The wound is then thoroughly irrigated using pulsatile lavage, and the wound is meticulously closed over a drain using absorbable, non-braided suture material. Treatment with 6 weeks of intravenous antibiotics as guided by an infectious disease consultant is standard in North America, followed typically by oral antibiotic treatment. Treatment with oral antibiotics can range from several weeks to lifelong, depending on the virulence of the infecting organism, the overall health of the patient, and the patient's ability to tolerate the oral antibiotic over an extended period of time. The decision to continue or discontinue antibiotic treatment is typically made with the input of the infectious disease consultant.

CASE 2: CHRONIC PERIPROSTHETIC INFECTION

History

A 68-year-old man presented 16 months following a primary THA, done at another hospital, with pain in

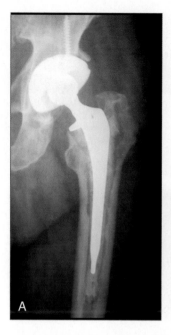
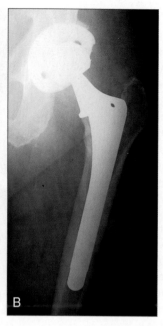

Figure 2   Radiographs of the hip of a 68-year-old man who presented with pain 16 months after a primary THA with a hybrid hip. **A,** Preoperative AP view demonstrates loosening of the cemented femoral component. **B,** Postoperative AP view demonstrates revision components in place following removal of the antibiotic-loaded cement spacer.

the surgical hip. Plain radiographs (**Figure 2, A**) showed a hybrid THA with loosening of the femoral component. The ESR was 99 mm/h (normal, 0 to 17 mm/h) and the CRP was 69 µg/mL (normal, 0 to 5 µg/mL). Based on the elevated laboratory test results and evidence of component loosening within 2 years of the index arthroplasty, an attempt was made to aspirate the hip; however, no fluid was obtained.

Case Management and Outcome

At the time of revision surgery, an intraoperative cell count showed 21,000 WBCs with 92% PMNs; the intraoperative frozen section was consistent with acute inflammation. The components were removed and an antibiotic-loaded spacer was fashioned using 3 g of vancomycin and 1.2 g of tobramycin per package of Palacos bone cement. Surgical cultures grew *S epidermidis* and *Streptococcus viridans*. The patient was treated with 6 weeks of intravenous antibiotics as guided by an infectious disease consultant. Antibiotics were then held for 3 weeks and the ESR and CRP were repeated; the ESR was 23 mm/h and the CRP was 7 µg/mL (both normal). The patient was returned to the operating room at 9 weeks following the resection arthroplasty. An intraoperative hip aspiration was performed; the synovial fluid WBC count was 240 with 57% PMNs. The frozen section showed scattered PMNs with foci of

up to 5 PMNs. Based on the overall picture of resolution of infection, the components were reimplanted (**Figure 2, B**) after a thorough débridement of the bony surfaces (including reaming of both the femur and acetabulum) and pulsatile lavage of the entire wound. Final surgical cultures were negative, and antibiotics were discontinued. At 4 years postoperatively, the patient is pain-free and the components show evidence of osseointegration.

Discussion

Recognizing the Problem and High-Risk Situations

In addition to the previously cited risk factors for acute postoperative infection, failure within 2 years of the index arthroplasty, a history of multiple prior surgeries, or revision surgery are particularly suggestive of infection.[6]

History and Physical Examination

Patients should be directly queried regarding prolonged drainage or antibiotic use at the time of the index arthroplasty and for a history of recent fever or infection that could have been associated with bacteremia (such as extraction of an infected tooth). Pain that is unrelated to activity, is constant, and that has been present since the time of surgery is likewise suggestive of infection. Prior skin incisions should be carefully inspected to identify active or healed sinus tracts or other evidence of delayed wound healing.

Laboratory Tests

An ESR and CRP should be ordered routinely in patients who present with a painful THA. Two studies have found that when both the ESR and CRP are normal, infection can be reliably ruled out.[2,7] If either of these values is elevated, infection should be suspected and further testing ordered. It is difficult to recommend specific maximum values, and in fact each laboratory defines its own normal ranges, but an ESR of >30 mm/h and a CRP of >10 mg/dL are commonly cited as abnormal.

Radiographs

Plain radiographs should be reviewed to identify implant loosening; serial radiographs are typically helpful in this regard. Evidence of rapid loosening in an otherwise well-executed reconstruction is particularly suggestive of infection (**Figure 2, A**).

Nuclear Medicine Studies

Nuclear medicine studies are not recommended for routine use in evaluating the painful and potentially infected THA because they are, in general, expensive, time-consuming, and not associated with adequate overall testing accuracy. Most surgeons use them on a selective basis when evaluating patients in whom surgery is not otherwise indicated and the diagnosis or etiology for a patient's pain is unclear.

Technetium-99 methylene diphosphonate bone scans can be useful in identifying subtle loosening; however, they cannot differentiate between septic and aseptic failure. Unfortunately, bone scans are sometimes abnormal for more than 1 year postoperatively, and in one study they were found to be no more helpful for identifying loosening than a careful review of serial plain radiographs.[8]

Gallium scans have been abandoned in most centers secondary to poor overall testing reliability.[9,10] Indium-111–labeled leukocyte scans have fallen into similar disfavor, although in one study[11] a negative result reliably ruled out infection with a negative predictive value of 95%. In an attempt to improve upon the high false-positive rate of indium scans, they have been combined with technetium-99m–labeled sulfur colloid marrow scanning to compensate for physiologic marrow packing. Unfortunately, this adds complexity and expense without substantially improving reliability.[12] More recently, positron emission tomography (PET) scanning has been advocated by one group;[13] however, PET scanning is costly. Data from additional centers will determine the ultimate utility of this tool.

Preoperative Joint Aspiration for Culture

The routine use of preoperative joint aspiration for culture before revision THA has been shown to be associated with a high rate of false-positive results.[14] Some authors have suggested a selective approach to preoperative aspiration, performing it only if laboratory values are suggestive of infection or if the implant has been in place for less than 5 years.[6] If a preoperative aspiration is performed, it is imperative that patients have been off antibiotics for at least 2 weeks and preferably 3 weeks before the aspiration to decrease the rate of false-negative results. More recent data from my institution suggest that an analysis of the synovial fluid WBC count is a much more reliable test. Optimal testing parameters were obtained by combining the ESR and CRP with the cell count. Early studies suggested a value of 50,000 WBC/mL as a criterion, but our study found the optimal cutoff value (as determined by using a receiver-operating curve) to be 3,000 WBC/mL when both the ESR and CRP were known to be elevated, or 9,000 WBC/mL if only one was elevated.[2]

Intraoperative Joint Aspiration

At my institution, after exposure of the joint capsule but before entering it, the hip joint is routinely aspirated and the aspirated fluid is sent for a synovial fluid WBC count and differential. As described above for preoperative joint aspiration, a recent analysis found this to be the best testing modality for predicting the presence or absence of infection. The result can usually be obtained within 30 minutes and yields an objective number that is easy to interpret. If the ESR and CRP were both elevated, the optimal cutoff value was 3,000 WBC/mL. If only one of the values was elevated, a WBC of 9,000 WBC/mL was required to accurately predict the presence of infection.[2]

Intraoperative Frozen Section Analysis

Intraoperative frozen section analysis has been shown to be a useful tool for the intraoperative identification of infection.[7,15] Unfortunately, this test requires a dedicated and interested pathologist (who may not be available at all centers), the results are both subjective and subject to sampling error, and the exact criteria for infection are not universally agreed upon. Most centers use an average of 10 PMNs present in the five most cellular fields,[16] but others have suggested that using an average of five provides better sensitivity.[17] The optimal tissue to be sampled includes the most suspicious-appearing areas of the joint capsule and the interfaces between the implant and the cement or the implant and the surrounding host bone. PMNs must be present in tissue (and not fibrin) to be counted for the analysis.

Intraoperative Gram Stains

Two separate studies have shown that intraoperative Gram stains have little value for diagnosing periprosthetic infection. Thus, the isolated use of this test is strongly discouraged, and the adjunctive use of an intraoperative Gram stain probably adds little to the overall clinical picture.[18,19]

Intraoperative Culture

If intraoperative cultures are to be obtained, most centers recommend obtaining three to five sets (including aerobic, anaerobic, fungal, and for acid-fast bacilli) because the rate of falsely positive cultures can be substantial.[20] In other cases, a patient may have all of the characteristics of infection, yet cultures are negative.[21] Culture swabs should be opened just before their use, handled carefully (taking care not to touch the swab itself with a gloved hand), and taken directly from around the implants themselves. Ultrasonification of the implants themselves has been shown to increase the yield of positive cultures, presumably decreasing the risk of false-negative results by releasing nonplanktonic bacteria from a protective slime that may make it difficult to definitively culture and identify them.[22]

Managing Chronic Periprosthetic Infection

Débridement

Débridement as a treatment modality for the chronically infected total hip is discouraged because the reported results are poor.[3]

Single-Stage Exchange

A direct, or "single-stage," exchange has been advocated for patients with an infected THA who are immunocomponent hosts (eg, nondiabetic, nonrheumatoid) with a known infecting organism that is of low virulence.[21] The technique was originally described using a cemented revision femoral component inserted with antibiotic-loaded cement. Although the technique never gained great popularity in North America, the trend toward diaphyseal-engaging, cementless femoral components has further decreased enthusiasm for this technique secondary to not only the loss of antibiotic-loaded cement, but also the morbidity of removal of a well-fixed stem if the infection is not eradicated and the difficulty of further reconstruction.

Two-Stage Exchange

A two-stage exchange protocol is standard treatment for an infected THA in North America. At the time of implant removal, the acetabulum is gently reamed with hemispherical reamers and the femur is reamed using flexible reamers. Experience at my institution shows that an extended trochanteric osteotomy can be safely used to remove well-fixed implants with primary fixation of the osteotomy leading to rapid healing if the soft-tissue attachments are respected.[23] A canal light is used to ensure that any cement present in the femoral canal is removed, and an intraoperative radiograph can be obtained if there is any doubt regarding complete hardware and cement removal.

Local antibiotic delivery is accomplished using bone cement that is hand-mixed with antibiotics. Palacos bone cement has been shown to have the best elution characteristics, and the combined use of antibiotics further improves elution. Although individual protocols vary at different institutions, 3 to 6 g of antibiotics are mixed with each package of cement; the most commonly used antibiotics are vancomycin and tobramycin.[24] Antibiotics are most commonly delivered as either a chain of beads or as a block placed into the acetabulum with a dowel of cement placed in the femur (**Figure 3, A**), as an articulating spacer that is either made as a mold (**Figure 3, B**) or fashioned by hand (**Figure 3, C**), or as part of the PROSTALAC (prosthesis with antibiotic-loaded acrylic cement) device (DePuy, Warsaw, IN)

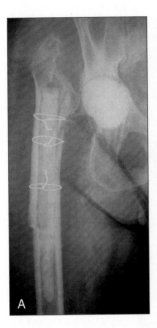 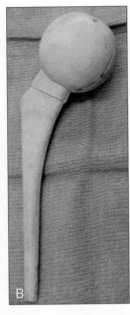 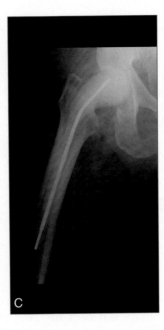 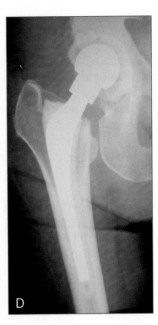

Figure 3 Options for local antibiotic delivery as part of a two-stage exchange for an infected THA. **A,** AP radiograph shows an antibiotic-loaded dowel of cement in the femur that was placed following removal of the infected femoral component. The extended osteotomy was closed with Luque wires, and additional antibiotic-loaded cement was placed into the acetabulum. **B,** Antibiotic-loaded cement spacer made with a mold (Stage One, Biomet, Warsaw, IN). **C,** Antibiotic-loaded cement spacer fashioned by hand over a threaded Steinmann pin. **D,** AP radiograph of an implanted PROSTALAC device shows the cemented femoral stem and cemented all-polyethylene acetabular component.

(**Figure 3, D**); however, the PROSTALAC device is not currently approved by the US Food and Drug Administration. Advantages of an articulating spacer include greater patient comfort and maintenance of leg length; this makes subsequent exposure at reimplantation easier and may decrease the risk of instability after reimplantation, because it is easier to restore leg length and offset. A nonarticulating spacer is chosen when acetabular bone stock loss is severe (eg, a Paprosky type III or higher acetabular defect); this increases the risk of further host-bone stock damage (because what remains is less supportive) and the risk of dislocation of the spacer because containment in a compromised acetabulum is more difficult to achieve.

In general, I prefer to use a nonbraided, absorbable suture for closure and do not use a drain. The patient is then typically treated with 6 weeks of organism-specific intravenous antibiotics as directed by the infectious disease consultant. Ideally, weekly ESR and CRP are obtained to observe the overall trend. The patient is seen 2 or 3 weeks following cessation of antibiotics, and the ESR and CRP are redrawn to assess whether the trend has continued or changed after antibiotic completion. Although there are few hard data to judge when the infection has been eradicated, decreasing laboratory values, healing of the wound, and a diminished pain pattern are all suggestive of infection resolution. At the time of reexploration, an intraoperative frozen section[25] is obtained, as is a synovial fluid WBC count with differential along with three to five full sets of cultures as described previously. After the antibiotic spacer is removed, all bony surfaces are meticulously cleared of fibrous tissue and reamed to expose fresh bleeding bone in the acetabulum, and, because my preference is for cementless femoral reconstruction, the canal is reamed with flexible reamers to débride the canal itself. The wound and all bony surfaces including the femoral canal are irrigated copiously using pulsatile lavage. If persistent infection is identified, a new spacer is placed; if there is evidence that the infection has resolved, I proceed with prosthesis reimplantation. The surgeon should be aware that second-stage reimplantations are notorious for developing postoperative instability, and the liberal use of large-diameter (36-mm or greater) femoral heads is recommended. Constrained liners are recommended for patients with abductor insufficiency.[26]

CASE 3: ACUTE HEMATOGENOUS INFECTION
History

A 66-year-old man reported to the emergency department 6 years following a primary THA. He had a history of fever and severe hip pain for 36 hours. The patient recently had sustained an injury by sliding down a ladder, severely abrading the anterior aspect of his knees and lower leg bilaterally. On physical examination, he was febrile to 102.1° and had large abrasions over the anterior aspect of both lower legs. An ESR and CRP were obtained; they were 102 mm/h and 137 µg/mL, respectively. Plain radiographs showed well-fixed cementless femoral and acetabular components (**Figure 4**). The hip was aspirated in the fluoroscopy suite and grossly purulent-appearing material was obtained; the cell count from the fluid showed 102,000 WBC/mL with 98% PMNs.

Case Management and Outcome

The patient was brought urgently to the operating room that evening, where an irrigation and débridement was performed along with exchange of the modular femoral head and polyethylene liner. At the time of surgery, the components were noted to be well fixed and in acceptable position. Surgical cultures showed *Bacteroides uniformis*. The patient was treated with intravenous antibiotics for 6 weeks as guided by an infectious disease specialist, followed by oral antibiotics for a year. At latest follow-up, the patient had been off antibiotics for more than 3 years and was asymptomatic with a normal ESR and CRP.

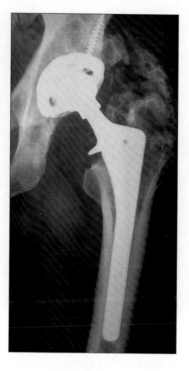

Figure 4 Preoperative AP radiograph of the hip of a 66-year-old man who presented 6 years after a primary THA with symptoms of acute fever and pain. The radiograph demonstrates well-fixed cementless components.

Discussion
Recognizing Acute Hematogenous Infection and High-Risk Situations

The diagnosis of an acute hematogenous infection following THA is most easily made in the patient who presents with an acute onset of hip pain (in the setting of a previously well-functioning THA) in conjunction with fever and a source of bacteremia. Patients seem to be at most risk in the first 2 years after surgery and are often immuncompromised (eg, a patient with rheumatoid arthritis who is on chronic steroid therapy). It is often difficult to determine precisely when the infection started, and the clinician should be wary of classifying an infection as acute hematogenous in a patient whose symptoms do not meet the criteria listed above, because chronic infections are far more common.

Managing Acute Hematogenous Infection

If an acute hematogenous infection is identified, the patient should be brought urgently to the operating room for irrigation and débridement as described above for an acute postoperative infection. Unfortunately, there is little literature available to guide the surgeon in terms of expected outcomes,[3,4] and often it is unclear whether an infection is truly acute hematogenous or chronic in nature. Although it seems reasonable to attempt irrigation and débridement for an acute hematogenous infection, débridement of a chronic infection routinely results in a treatment failure. When the diagnosis is unclear, the patient should be educated regarding this dilemma and given the option of a two-stage exchange as well as an irrigation and débridement. Surgical débridement is followed by a 6-week course of intravenous antibiotics and oral antibiotics for at least 1 year and in some cases life-long, depending on the patient's ability to tolerate long-term oral antibiotic therapy.

STRATEGIES TO MINIMIZE COMMON COMPLICATIONS

Acute Postoperative Infection

The routine administration of prophylactic antibiotics before the skin incision is imperative to decrease the risk of surgical-site infection. Even in revision cases, a recent study showed that in patients with a known infection, the use of antibiotics before the skin incision did not compromise culture accuracy.[27] The most commonly used antibiotic in the United States is cefazolin, which should be administered within 1 hour of the surgical incision. Dosage is 1 g for patients who weigh less than 80 kg and 2 g for those over 80 kg. In patients with a known allergy to cefazolin or penicillin, vancomycin or clindamycin is recommended. Additional factors that may lower the risk of acute postoperative infection include the use of laminar air flow (particularly vertical laminar air flow), the use of body exhaust suits, decreasing operating room traffic, and the use of ultraviolet light.

If an acute postoperative infection is suspected, the indiscriminate use of oral antibiotics is strongly discouraged as this may mask a deep infection that requires surgical débridement. If surgical débridement is undertaken, the use of vancomycin is recommended until final surgical culture results are known because, as a study of 146 infected total joint arthroplasties showed, it will cover the most likely infecting organisms.[28] One factor that is unclear is how to precisely define an acute postoperative infection; however, an infection that develops beyond 6 weeks postoperatively should probably be managed as a chronic infection.

Chronic Periprosthetic Infection

If a chronic infection is diagnosed, key factors in management include avoiding surgical débridement with component retention, performing a thorough surgical débridement, removing all retained components and cement, and involving an infectious disease specialist to assist with antibiotic management. If the infecting organism is not known preoperatively, antibiotic coverage with vancomycin should be used until final culture results are known.[28]

Acute Hematogenous Infection

The most common pitfall when addressing an acute hematogenous infection is mistaking a chronic infection for one that is acute hematogenous in nature; the clinician should be wary of this potential. Patients should be educated about the risks of acute hematogenous infection and the importance of prophylactic antibiotic use before invasive medical or dental procedures throughout their lifetime. Official American Academy of Orthopaedic Surgeons and American Dental Association guidelines include the prophylactic use of amoxicillin clavulanate, 2 g orally, 1 hour before routine dental work (or clindamycin in patients with a penicillin allergy) for the first 2 years postoperatively, although some surgeons recommend antibiotic treatment before even routine dental work for the patient's entire life. Further, patients should be instructed that any systemic, bacterial illness must be treated aggressively and that if pain develops in the replaced joint, the operating surgeon's office should be contacted immediately for evaluation and possible treatment.

REFERENCES

1. Patel VP, Walsh M, Sehgal B, Preston C, DeWal H, Di Cesare PE: Factors associated with prolonged wound drainage after primary total hip and knee arthroplasty. *J Bone Joint Surg Am* 2007;89:33-38.

2. Schinsky M, Della Valle CJ, Sporer SM, Paprosky WG: Perioperative testing for joint infection in patients undergoing revision total hip arthroplasty. *J Bone Joint Surg Am* 2008;9: 1869-1875.

3. Crockarell JR, Hanssen AD, Osmon DR, Morrey BF: Treatment of infection with debridement and retention of the components following hip arthroplasty. *J Bone Joint Surg Am* 1998;80:1306-1312.

4. Tsukayama DT, Estrada R, Gustilo RB: Infection after total hip arthroplasty: A study of the treatment of one hundred and six infections. *J Bone Joint Surg Am* 1996;78:512-523.

5. Hanssen AD, Rand JA: Evaluation and treatment of infection at the site of a total hip or knee arthroplasty. *Instr Course Lect* 1999; 48:111-122.

6. Lachiewicz PF, Rogers GD, Thomason HC: Aspiration of the hip joint before revision total hip arthroplasty: Clinical and laboratory factors influencing attainment of a positive culture. *J Bone Joint Surg Am* 1996;78:749-754.

7. Spangehl MJ, Masri BA, O'Connell JX, Duncan CP: Prospective analysis of preoperative and intraoperative investigations for the diagnosis of infection at the sites of two hundred and two revision total hip arthroplasties. *J Bone Joint Surg Am* 1999;81:672-683.

8. Lieberman JR, Huo MH, Schneider R, Salvati EA, Rodi S: Evaluation of painful hip arthroplasties: Are technetium bone scans necessary? *J Bone Joint Surg Br* 1993;75:475-478.

9. Kraemer WJ, Saplys R, Waddell JP, Morton J: Bone scan, gallium scan, and hip aspiration in the diagnosis of infected total hip arthroplasty. *J Arthroplasty* 1993;8:611-616.

10. Merkel KD, Brown ML, Dewanjee MK, Fitzgerald RH Jr: Comparison of indium-labeled-leukocyte imaging with sequential technetium-gallium scanning in the diagnosis of low-grade musculoskeletal sepsis: A prospective study. *J Bone Joint Surg Am* 1985;67:465-476.

11. Scher DM, Pak K, Lonner JH, Finkel JE, Zuckerman JD, Di Cesare PE: The predictive value of indium-111 leukocyte scans in the diagnosis of infected total hip, knee, or resection arthroplasties. *J Arthroplasty* 2000;15:295-300.

12. Joseph TN, Mujtaba M, Chen AL, et al: Efficacy of combined technetium-99m sulfur colloid/indium-111 leukocyte scans to detect infected total hip and knee arthroplasties. *J Arthroplasty* 2001;16:753-758.

13. Pill SG, Parvizi J, Tang PH, et al: Comparison of fluorodeoxyglucose positron emission tomography and (111)indium-white blood cell imaging in the diagnosis of periprosthetic infection of the hip. *J Arthroplasty* 2006;21(6 Suppl 2):91-97.

14. Barrack RL, Harris WH: The value of aspiration of the hip joint before revision total hip arthroplasty. *J Bone Joint Surg Am* 1993;75:66-76.

15. Lonner JH, Desai P, Dicesare PE, Steiner G, Zuckerman JD: The reliability of analysis of intraoperative frozen sections for identifying active infection during revision hip or knee arthroplasty. *J Bone Joint Surg Am* 1996;78:1553-1558.

16. Feldman DS, Lonner JH, Desai P, Zuckerman JD: The role of intraoperative frozen sections in revision total joint arthroplasty. *J Bone Joint Surg Am* 1995;77:1807-1813.

17. Mirra JM, Marder RA, Amstutz HC: The pathology of failed total joint arthroplasty. *Clin Orthop Relat Res* 1982;170:175-183.

18. Della Valle CJ, Scher DM, Kim YH, et al: The role of intraoperative Gram stain in revision total joint arthroplasty. *J Arthroplasty* 1999;14:500-504.

19. Spangehl MJ, Masterson E, Masri BA, O'Connell JX, Duncan CP: The role of intraoperative gram stain in the diagnosis of infection during revision total hip arthroplasty. *J Arthroplasty* 1999;14:952-956.

20. Padgett DE, Silverman A, Sachjowicz F, Simpson RB, Rosenberg AG, Galante JO: Efficacy of intraoperative cultures obtained during revision total hip arthroplasty. *J Arthroplasty* 1995;10:420-426.

21. Buchholz HW, Elson RA, Engelbrecht E, Lodenkamper H, Rottger J, Siegel A: Management of deep infection of total hip replacement. *J Bone Joint Surg Br* 1981;63:342-353.

22. Trampuz A, Piper KE, Jacobson MJ, et al: Sonication of removed hip and knee prostheses for diagnosis of infection. *N Engl J Med* 2007;357:654-663.

23. Levine B, Della Valle CJ, Hamming M, Sporer S, Berger RA, Paprosky W: Use of the extended trochanteric osteotomy in treating prosthetic hip infection. *J Arthroplasty* 2008; epub ahead of print.

24. Joseph TN, Chen AL, Di Cesare PE: Use of antibiotic-impregnated

cement in total joint arthroplasty. *J Am Acad Orthop Surg* 2003;11:38-47.

25. Della Valle CJ, Bogner E, Desai P, et al: Analysis of frozen sections of intraoperative specimens obtained at the time of reoperation after hip or knee resection arthroplasty for the treatment of infection. *J Bone Joint Surg Am* 1999;81:684-689.

26. Kung PL, Ries MD: Effect of femoral head size and abductors on dislocation after revision THA. *Clin Orthop Relat Res* 2007;465:170-174.

27. Ghanem E, Parvizi J, Clohisy J, Burnett S, Sharkey PF, Barrack R: Perioperative antibiotics should not be withheld in proven cases of periprosthetic infection. *Clin Orthop Relat Res* 2007;461:44-47.

28. Fulkerson E, Della Valle CJ, Wise B, Walsh M, Preston C, Di Cesare PE: Antibiotic susceptibility of bacteria infecting total joint arthroplasty sites. *J Bone Joint Surg Am* 2006;88:1231-1237.

Chapter 7

WEAR AND OSTEOLYSIS

David Manning, MD
*Joshua J. Jacobs, MD

CASE 1: LYSIS IN YOUNG, ACTIVE TOTAL HIP ARTHROPLASTY PATIENTS

History

A 43-year-old woman presented for evaluation of painless shortening of the left lower extremity 9 years after a left total hip arthroplasty (THA) performed for osteonecrosis. The patient did not describe limited range of motion, limp, or decreased ambulatory capacity. Her Harris hip score was 98, and her University of California at Los Angeles (UCLA) activity score was 8 (scale, 1 to 10). Review of the prior surgical notes indicated that the implants used for her THA were a cementless APR II-T cup and stem (Intermedics Orthopedics, Austin, TX) and a 28-mm zirconia femoral head articulating with conventional polyethylene. The patient had not been seen since her first postoperative visit and thus had not had routine surveillance radiographs performed.

Current Problem

Initial evaluation included a history, physical examination, and radiographs. Specific questions were asked to elicit the initial diagnosis and symptoms, the progress of initial wound healing, any suggestion of infection, postoperative activity, and whether the patient had regular follow-up. The patient had an original diagnosis of osteonecrosis and an uneventful postoperative course; however, there was no routine follow-up.

The physical examination focused on the neurovascular status of the extremity, the location of the prior incision, and any signs of wound healing problems, abductor power, range of motion, and limb length. The patient was noted to have a posterior hip incision with good abductor power, no stiffness,

*Joshua J. Jacobs, MD, or the department with which he is affiliated has received research or institutional support from Zimmer, Wright Medical, Medtronic, Spinal Motion, Archus, and Advanced Spine Technology and is a consultant for or an employee of Zimmer, Wright Medical, and Medtronic.

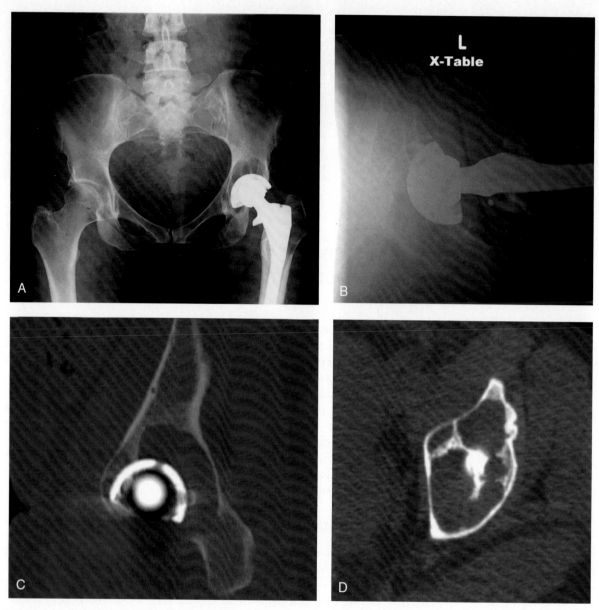

Figure 1   Images of the 43-year-old woman with osteolysis following THA described in Case 1. **A,** AP pelvic radiograph depicting type I shell and stable femoral component 9 years after THA with expansile osteolysis of the pelvis, proximal femoral stress-shielding, and greater trochanteric osteolysis. Acetabular shell inclination angle is 42°. **B,** Shoot-through hip radiograph suggests an anteverted acetabular shell and expansile lysis of posterior column. **C,** Axial CT scan shows severe dome osteolysis. **D,** Coronal CT scan shows large posterior column lysis around acetabular shell screw holes.

and relatively equal limb lengths. Radiographs (including an AP pelvis, Judet views, AP and lateral views of the hip, as well as a cross-table lateral) indicated stable cementless femoral and acetabular implants in acceptable position with near polyethylene wear-through and expansile osteolysis of the pelvis (**Figure 1**). Modest proximal femoral stress-shielding and greater trochanteric osteolysis were noted around the femoral prosthesis. Radiographic and implant record data yielded classification of the shell as type I. The patient was instructed to curtail her activities, and revision surgery was planned.

Discussion

Recognizing the Problem and High-Risk Situations

Osteolysis and late aseptic implant failure is a major concern with regard to the long-term survival of THA.[1-3] Osteolysis-related implant loosening represents the single most common complication of total joint arthroplasties and is estimated to occur in more than 25% of all implant recipients.[3] The incidence of osteolysis in THA may be as high as 40% at 10 years of follow-up.[3] Osteolysis is understood to be a cell-mediated inflammatory response to prosthesis wear–related particle debris.[1-4] Various cytokines, receptor activator of nuclear factor κ B ligand, and osteoprotegrin act in both autocrine and paracrine fashions to unlink bone formation and bone resorption in the peri-implant environment. The result is a relative decrease in osteoblast activity, a relative increase in osteoclast differentiation and activity, as well as an increase in fibroblast activity. Ultimately, peri-implant bone is resorbed, and inflammatory fibrous tissue fills the bone voids.[4]

Osteolysis is typically painless and therefore clinically silent. Pain routinely occurs only in association with implant loosening or periprosthetic fracture. Detection of osteolysis before implant loosening or periprosthetic fracture occurs is only possible with routine radiographic surveillance. Several risk factors for wear and osteolysis exist and may be considered under the broader headings of patient-related factors, implant-related factors, surgical factors, and bearing-related factors.

Patient-Related Risk Factors

Age, sex, and activity level all have been linked to accelerated wear in patients undergoing THA with conventional polyethylene bearings. In a study of the influence of demographic and technical variables on the incidence of osteolysis in Charnley primary low-friction hip arthroplasty, Nercessian and associates[5] found that younger patients (age <65 years) and men were both found to have higher wear rates and a significantly increased incidence of osteolysis ($P < 0.05$). Joshi and associates[6] noted that in patients undergoing Charnley primary low-friction hip arthroplasty, high rates of wear, component instability, and osteolysis were three times more common in men than in women. The amount of acetabular liner wear is a function of the femoral head distance traveled against the bearing counterpart over time. It is assumed that gender and age are surrogate markers for patient activity and, in turn, distance traveled by the femoral head. Although joint reaction force and therefore bearing stress are affected by patient weight or body mass index, neither has been conclusively linked to increased wear.[7]

The link between wear and osteolysis is predicated on the assumption that increased wear (particle generation) results in more osteolysis. Indeed, increased true wear is significantly associated with osteolysis at 10 years after the operation; however, the relationship between wear and osteolysis is not linear. In a study of 48 THAs at minimum 10-year follow-up, Dowd and associates[8] demonstrated that osteolysis was strongly associated with increasing true wear rates ($P <0.001$). Osteolysis developed in 0% of hips with a true wear rate of less than 0.1 mm per year, in 43% of hips with a rate between 0.1 and 0.2 mm per year, in 80% of hips with a rate between 0.2 and 0.3 mm per year, and in 100% of hips with a rate of greater than 0.3 mm per year.[8] Osteolysis, although clearly linked to the generation of prosthetic debris, is multifactorial and includes the variability of individual patients' biologic response to debris.[4]

In the case presented here, the patient was 34 years of age at the time of original arthroplasty. The patient also reported observing no limitations in activity and presented with a UCLA activity score of 8. Patient age and activity are likely related to poor bearing performance in this case.

Implant-Related Factors

Several implant-related factors have been linked to wear and osteolysis and are highlighted by some of the early experience with cementless THA. High wear rates and specific design parameters of the porous-coated anatomic (PCA; Osteonics, Mahwah, NJ) and the Harris-Galante (HG; Zimmer, Inc,

Warsaw, IN) prostheses resulted in high rates of osteolysis.[9] The PCA is a cobalt-chrome beaded device with circumferential porous coating on the femoral component; the acetabular shell is equipped with two beaded prongs intended to aid in initial fixation by engaging the superior-outer aspect of the bony acetabulum. Long-term follow-up of this device is commonly associated with vertically implanted shells and elevated wear rates (abduction angle >55° often is necessary to engage beaded prongs).[9] High abduction angles increase bearing stress and bearing wear. In the PCA system, osteolysis is common peripherally in pelvic zones 1 and 3 as well as femoral zones 1 and 7.[9] The HG total hip is a titanium fiber metal device with patch porous coating on the femoral side and multiple screw holes in the acetabular shell. The acetabular shell is equipped with a first-generation polyethylene locking mechanism that allows micromotion and backside wear potential. Long-term follow-up of this device is associated with expansile osteolysis in all pelvic zones and osteolysis in femoral zones distal to the porous coating.[9,10] At retrieval analysis, the polyethylene liner displays backside material loss and cold flow at the screw holes. As an aggregate, these early experiences prove that circumferential porous coating on the femoral side eliminates distal femoral osteolysis, that poor polyethylene locking mechanisms allow unintended wear modes to occur, and that acetabular screw holes allow increased particle access to periacetabular bone. The culmination of these observations and conclusions is the concept of the effective joint space, as reported by Schmalzried and associates[11] in 1992. In addition to bearing modifications, contemporary prostheses include circumferential porous coating of the femoral component, no-hole acetabular shell options, monoblock acetabular implant options, improved polyethylene locking mechanisms for modular systems, and, in some cases, a polished inner surface of the acetabular shell.

The femoral component used in the case presented here is circumferentially porous coated and successfully prevents distal femoral osteolysis. The acetabular component has multiple screw holes and a modest locking mechanism. Bearing micromotion and backside wear occurred, and the multiple screw holes allowed particulate debris to gain access to

peri-implant bone. The result was expansile osteolysis of the pelvis (**Figure 1**).

Surgical Factors

The PCA experience aptly outlines the negative effect of high acetabular abduction angle on wear and osteolysis.[9,12] This finding has been reproduced by other investigators in other implant systems as well. Most recently, Patil and associates[12] reported that an abduction angle greater than 50° was associated with increased linear and volumetric polyethylene wear in a series of patients receiving cementless devices with conventional polyethylene. The authors further identified that failure to restore femoral offset to within 4 mm of anatomic alignment increased linear and volumetric wear as well.[12] These findings may be interpreted to suggest continued adherence to Charnley's original idea of a low-friction arthroplasty. Restoration of hip center, medialization of the acetabular component, abduction less than 50°, restoration of femoral offset, and restoration of hip length all contribute to decreasing the joint reactive force and bearing stress. Bearing wear is likely to be minimized in this low-stress environment. In addition, surgeons should be alerted to the potential for particle generation via unintended wear modes (third-body wear from retained bone or cement particles) and unintended wear sites (femoral neck or head skirt impingement with an improperly positioned acetabular component or a lipped/face-changing liner).

In the case presented here, the acetabular component is appropriately abducted and anteverted. The femoral offset and length, before bearing wear, is equal to that of the contralateral hip. The hip center is slightly lateralized (the acetabular shell is not seated against the medial wall), resulting in increased body moment arm, joint reactive force, and bearing stress (**Figure 1**).

Bearing Factors

Osteolysis, once termed "cement disease," is now known to be induced by any particulate biomaterial smaller than 10 μm.[4] The usual source for generating biomaterial particles in this size range after THA is the bearing. Osteolysis is common after THA using conventional polyethylene. Modern bearing choices (highly cross-linked polyethylene (HXLPE), ceramic-on-ceramic, and metal-on-metal) represent an evolution intended to combat wear and osteolysis. In their current forms, at short- to midterm follow-up, there is little evidence linking modern bearing surfaces, osteolysis, and aseptic loosening. Modern bearings are now routinely used as prophylaxis against osteolysis. However, each modern bearing choice has potential shortcomings.

Ultra-High Molecular Weight Polyethylene

Conventional ultra-high molecular weight polyethylene (UHMWPE) bearings are inextricably linked to wear and osteolysis. One key factor in the performance of polyethylene is its potential to oxidize. In an oxygen-rich environment, polyethylene may undergo surface and subsurface oxidation, resulting in altered mechanical properties and wear performance. Newer procedures dramatically reduce oxidation during the sterilization and storage of the bearing by simply limiting exposure to oxygen. However, polyethylene that has retained free radicals by virtue of exposure to gamma irradiation (even in the absence of oxygen exposure during sterilization and storage) has been shown to oxidize in vivo.

Experience with conventional polyethylene products has shed light on the wear effects of differing bar stock, processing techniques (machining versus molding), and sterilization methods (ethylene oxide, gas plasma, and gamma irradiation). The effects of each are beyond the scope of this chapter, but the effects of polyethylene thickness, femoral head type, and size on wear deserve special attention. Modular polyethylene bearings less than 6 to 7 mm in nominal thickness are associated with increased wear rates and failure.[13] Femoral head size is inversely proportional to linear wear rate and directly proportional to volumetric wear rate.[13,14] Osteolysis is most closely related to volumetric wear rates.[14] Therefore, when small, modular acetabular shells and conventional polyethylene bearings are used, consideration should be given to decreasing head size and maximizing polyethylene thickness. Untreated titanium counter bearings should not be used because they are relatively soft and prone to scratching and abrasive wear.

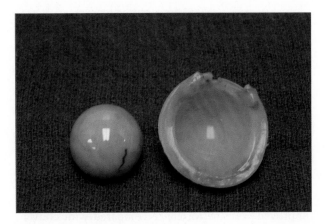

Figure 2 On the left, retrieved zirconia femoral ball with metal staining from bearing wear-through at the rim. On the right, retrieved conventional polyethylene liner with evidence of wear, oxidation, and cracking. Near wear-through is evidenced by blue hue from background seen at the pole.

Individual study results vary, and controversy persists regarding the choice of cobalt-chrome versus ceramic counter bearing.

In the case presented here, a 46-mm modular acetabular shell with polyethylene sterilized and packaged in an oxygen-free environment was mated with a 28-mm zirconia ceramic counter bearing. The resultant polyethylene thickness is 7 mm at the dome. At retrieval, the bearing was visibly worn, with oxidation and surface cracking (**Figure 2**).

Highly Cross-Linked Polyethylene

The process of cross-linking UHMWPE involves irradiating the material (with gamma rays or an electron beam) to induce chemical cross-links in the amorphous zones of the polymer. Cross-links make the material more resistant to wear and multidirectional shear forces.[15] The degree of cross-linking and wear resistance is related to radiation dose in a nonlinear fashion.[15]

Gamma irradiation also creates free radicals in the amorphous zones of the polymer.[15] In an oxygen-rich environment, those free radicals will undergo oxidation and decay similar to non–highly cross-linked polyethylenes. Product-specific methods of eliminating free radicals (eg, melting, annealing) are used to deter oxidation but are associated with decreased mechanical properties of the material. In general,

HXLPEs have a lower fatigue failure strength and greater fatigue crack propagation than non–highly cross-linked polyethylenes.[15] The resultant highly cross-linked products provide a balance between improved wear resistance and altered mechanical properties. Although mechanical failures have been reported, they typically have been associated with malpositioned (particularly vertical) implants.

In vitro wear analyses of 10-Mrad HXLPE show negligible wear at more than 30 million cycles on the Boston hip simulator.[15] Early and midterm in vivo evaluation of these materials confirm 60% to 90% improved wear performance compared with conventional polyethylene.[16] Osteolysis has not been reported at short- to midterm follow-up of 10-Mrad HXLPE.[16]

Ceramic-on-Ceramic Bearings

Contemporary ceramic-on-ceramic bearings provide a hard, scratch-resistant, and hydrophilic bearing couple with reduced wear and reduced particle generation.[17] Early iterations of this bearing were sometimes associated with high loosening rates, bearing fracture rates as high as 13%, and isolated cases of accelerated wear.[17] Aseptic loosening of older ceramic THAs may be attributable to non-bearing factors such as poor implant design and fixation methods.[17,18] High bearing fracture rates of early designs are attributable to manufacturing issues such as inconsistent ceramic grain size and processing.[17,18] Modern ceramic bearings are generated using hot isostatic pressing of highly pure, small-grain ceramics. Although bearing fracture is still a concern, fracture rates of ceramic femoral heads manufactured using these techniques are estimated to be 4 in 100,000.[17,18]

The hydrophilic nature of ceramic improves the wettability of the material and yields improved joint lubricity.[17] Linear wear rates of approximately 1 μm per year have been reported in hip simulator studies using bovine serum as a lubricant.[17] Although ceramic particles are biologically active and may be ingested by macrophages, the particle load to surrounding tissues associated with such low wear rates is not likely to induce osteolysis. Concerns still exist for metal staining and atypical wear patterns (stripe wear), but the clinical significance is unclear. One clinical problem with ceramic bearings gaining new exposure is the so-called "squeaking hip." Audible squeaks in ceramic-on-ceramic bearings have been reported in up to 9% of patients and have led to revision surgery in severe cases.[19]

Metal-on-Metal Bearings

Early iterations of metal-on-metal bearing THAs were associated with high acetabular loosening rates and isolated cases of accelerated wear.[20] Aseptic loosening of the early McKee-Farrar metal-on-metal THA was attributable to suboptimal metallurgy, manufacturing, bearing tolerance, and bony fixation. Nevertheless, there are some reports of excellent long-term survivorship of the McKee-Farrar compared with the Charnley low-friction arthroplasty. Brown and associates[21] reported 84% survivorship in 129 patients at 20-year follow-up, with Kaplan-Meier survivorship of 74% at 28 years. In another review of the survivorship of the McKee-Farrar metal-on-metal THA, Jacobsson and associates[22] report 77% survivorship at 20 years in contrast to 73% survivorship for the Charnley THA during the same follow-up period. Osteolysis was rarely observed during long-term follow-up of patients having metal-on-metal THA, in contrast with that of Charnley low-friction arthroplasty.[21,22] Subsequent improvements have been made on all fronts in contemporary metal-on-metal designs, but many of the same questions remain. Simultaneously, new questions about metal ion release and metal hypersensitivity have arisen.

Elevated levels of cobalt and chromium in serum and metal particles in the reticuloendothelial system (liver, spleen, periaortic lymph nodes) have been identified in patients receiving metal-on-metal hips.[23] The physiologic effects of elevated ion levels are unknown. A retrospective analysis by Visuri and associates[24] examined the risk of carcinoma, sarcoma, and myeloplastic disease in McKee-Farrar and conventional metal-on-polyethylene THA. No statistically significant difference was identified in the incidence of cancer in the patients with metal-on-metal implants present for more than 20 years.[24] Other population-based surveys have concluded similar findings. However, given the long latency (>20 years) for metal-induced carcinogenesis and the relatively small sample sizes (measured in person-years) studied, this issue has yet to be resolved.

Metal hypersensitivity in patients with metal-on-metal THAs as a correlation between in vitro lymphocyte reactivity and serum cobalt levels has been demonstrated.[25,26] Histologically, the presence of perivascular lymphocytic infiltrates in the pseudocapsule of some patients undergoing revision of metal-on-metal hip arthroplasties is significantly different than the histiocytic response observed in patients with polyethylene wear.[27] This finding suggests a type IV immune response in this subset of patients. Metal sensitivity may be responsible for the reported linear radiolucencies around some previously well-fixed cementless acetabular components in metal-on-metal THAs and may represent a new mode of implant failure.[28]

Patient Evaluation

Osteolysis alone is rarely painful; by the time the patient is symptomatic, the destruction of periprosthetic bone may be extensive. Radiologic signs of implant failure may precede clinical symptoms by months to several years.[29] Regular clinical and radiographic follow-up care is generally recommended, even for asymptomatic patients. In 1995, the National Institutes of Health issued a statement on THA and concluded that continued periodic follow-up is necessary to identify early evidence of impending failure so as to permit remedial actions before a catastrophic event.[30]

In 2003, a survey of 682 active American Association of Hip and Knee Surgeons (AAHKS) members attempted to identify what type of follow-up care (clinical examination, with or without radiographs, and outcome questionnaires) they recommended.[31] Scheduled clinical examinations with review of radiographs by an orthopaedist were recommended by 95.9% of respondents. Different follow-up patterns were identified over the lifetime of an implant. In the early postoperative period (1 to 5 years), annual or biannual follow-up evaluations were most common (annual, 45.9%; biannual, 39.5%). In the midterm (6 to 10 years), biannual care was predominant (50.1%). After 10 years, recommendations for annual (37.3%) or biannual (42.9%) follow-up evaluations were again more evenly split. The most common reason for increasing the frequency of evaluation related directly to clinical or radiographic signs of actual or potential failure

(93.5%).[31] The results show a consistent, high level of agreement among AAHKS members that THA patients should be followed with clinical and radiographic examinations at regular intervals.

Nonsurgical Management

Several classes of potential modulators of bone homeostasis (nonsteroidal anti-inflammatory drugs and cyclooxygenase-2 inhibitors, bisphosphonates, tumor necrosis factor-α, and osteoprotegrin) have been postulated to offer benefit in the treatment of osteolysis.[32] In vitro and animal data support the continued investigation of several available medications; however, the low toxicity and widespread applicability of bisphosphonates make this class of drugs attractive for the potential treatment of periprosthetic osteolysis.

Several in vitro and animal studies report that bisphosphonates reduce osteoclastic bone resorption.[32] Unfortunately, few clinical data are available that support the efficacy of bisphosphonates in preventing osteolysis in humans. One clinical study has shown that alendronate can reduce the periprosthetic bone loss that develops soon after THA.[33] However, as the authors of that study pointed out, this early bone loss is probably secondary to stress shielding rather than to wear debris–induced osteolysis. Rubash and associates[34] performed a randomized multicenter clinical trial to evaluate the effect of alendronate on the radiographic progression of osteolytic lesions. After 18 months, no effect on lesion size was appreciated.[34] The poor sensitivity of plain radiographs in detecting subtle changes in lesion size may explain the lack of effect, but the findings do not support the routine use of alendronate in the treatment of osteolysis.

Surgical Management

Surgery remains the primary mode of management of osteolysis after THA and is indicated when patient evaluation detects implant loosening, bearing wear-through, impending failure, or severe bone loss. In patients who have received regular follow-up evaluation, osteolysis is generally detected before implant failure or major structural bone loss. In such cases, surgery may be planned electively before failure to effect a change that may result in retention of well-fixed components.

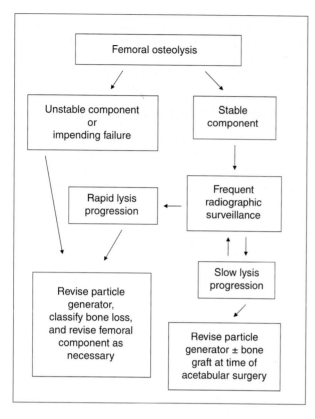

Figure 3 Algorithm for the management of femoral osteolysis.

Lysis of the femur around circumferentially porous-coated and cemented components is usually limited to the proximal femur and does not threaten implant stability. In such cases, retention of the component with bone grafting of proximal cavitary defects is generally undertaken. When the component is loose, revision is necessary in addition to management of bone loss. A femoral bone stock and implant management algorithm is presented in **Figure 3**. Care is necessary to prevent iatrogenic fracture of the greater trochanter during revision surgery because it is subject to the effects of both osteolysis and stress shielding.

The more common scenario is pelvic osteolysis with bearing wear. Osteolysis with bearing wear and loosening of the metal shell necessitates revision arthroplasty. However, the surgeon frequently must decide whether to remove a well-fixed porous-coated socket when reoperating for osteolysis and polyethylene wear. One strategy is to remove the well-fixed socket, graft defects, and revise the sock-et. This approach is associated with damage to the acetabular bone when removing a well-fixed cementless socket. Iatrogenic bone loss in addition to osteolytic bone loss may create a difficult revision scenario that challenges implant fixation techniques. A second strategy involves liner exchange and débridement with bone grafting of osteolytic lesions. Maloney and associates[35] reviewed their experience with revision surgery of well-fixed cementless acetabular components, and the results of socket removal were compared with results of liner exchange. Sixty-eight well-fixed acetabular cups with osteolysis and polyethylene wear were subdivided based on whether the shell was retained, the liner was exchanged, and débridement with or without bone grafting of osteolytic lesions was performed (type I case) or the socket was removed and a complete revision performed (type II case). In 40 type I cases, the polyethylene liner was exchanged and the osteolytic lesions were débrided. Allograft bone chips were used to graft the lytic defect in 29 patients; in the remaining 11 patients, the lesions were débrided but not grafted. In 28 type II cases, the socket was revised. At final follow-up, all of the acetabular components were radiographically stable and no new osteolytic lesions were identified. In the 40 type I cases, approximately one third of the lesions had resolved completely, regardless of whether they were grafted. The remaining two thirds of the lesions decreased in size. Both strategies were successful in halting the process of osteolysis at a mean follow-up of 3.5 years. However, removal of well-fixed sockets was associated with significantly more bone loss as evidenced by the large increase in revision cup size. The average diameter of the sockets removed was 52 mm, whereas the average diameter of the sockets implanted was 66 mm.[35]

Well-fixed metal porous-coated shells in the setting of bearing wear and osteolysis have been classified for the purpose of directing patient management (**Table 1**).[35,36] Briefly, in a type I shell, the metal porous-coated shell is radiographically stable and the polyethylene liner is modular. Bearing exchange and osteolysis débridement with or without grafting is the procedure of choice if the following conditions are met: (1) the cup is well positioned (to optimize both wear and stability), (2) the

TABLE 1 Acetabular Implant Classification for Decision Making in the Management of Periprosthetic Pelvic Osteolysis

Acetabular Shell Class	Characteristics

Type I	Stable and all of the following:
	  Well-positioned modular implant
	  Good track record
	  Undamaged shell
	  Intact/suitable locking mechanism*
	  Polyethylene liner adequate thickness

Type II	Stable and one of the following:
	  Poorly positioned implant
	  Nonmodular implant
	  Poor track record
	  Damaged implant
	  Unsuitable locking mechanism
	  Minimum thickness polyethylene not available

Type III	Radiographically loose

*In cases of shell with damaged or unsuitable locking mechanism but otherwise type I, cementing a new liner is an acceptable option. (Data from Rubash HE, Sinha RK, Paprosky W, Engh CA, Maloney WJ: A new classification system for the management of acetabular osteolysis after total hip arthroplasty. Instr Course Lect 1999;48:37-42.)

locking mechanism for the modular acetabular component is intact, (3) the polyethylene liner replacement is of adequate thickness, (4) the implant has an acceptable track record of survivorship, and (5) the metal shell is not damaged iatrogenically or from bearing wear-through.[35,36] One caveat in the type I shell scenario includes the option to cement a liner into a well-fixed shell with a damaged locking mechanism. The use of HXLPE is preferred when revising conventional polyethylene in a type I shell. Surprising morbidity is associated with isolated bearing exchange, with dislocation reportedly occurring in up to 25% of cases;[37] thus, thought should be given to using larger-size femoral heads (if polyethylene thickness is judged to be adequate). Great care must be taken intraoperatively to test and optimize stability, including a search for sources of impingement and meticulous soft-tissue capsular repair.[38] Surgical approach also may be important, with anterior and anterolateral approaches recommended by some surgeons (as opposed to a posterior approach) for isolated head and liner exchanges.

In a type II shell, the metal shell is radiographically stable. However, the implant fails to meet the six criteria for retention, and the well-fixed socket is removed; specialized curved osteotomes (specifically sized to the outer diameter of the metal shell) have made removal of well-fixed shells more technically straightforward. Reasons for removing a well-fixed socket include malposition, damage to the metal shell, a damaged or poor locking mechanism, inability to provide a polyethylene replacement liner of adequate thickness, and poor implant track record for survivorship. In a type III shell, there is radiographic evidence of a loose cup, and component revision is necessary.[35,36] This classification has been incorporated into the acetabular management algorithm in **Figure 4**.

Case Management and Outcome

In our case of a 43-year-old woman 9 years after THA, revision surgery was performed via a posterior surgical approach. Intraoperatively, stability and appropriate position of the cementless compo-

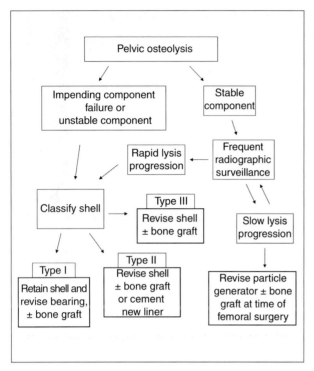

Figure 4 Algorithm for the management of pelvic osteolysis.

nents were confirmed, and the components were retained. The modular femoral head and acetabular liner were removed, and the pelvic osteolytic lesion was débrided through the screw holes in the shell, irrigated with pulsatile lavage, and grafted with 120 mL of fresh-frozen cancellous allograft bone. The greater trochanter was débrided proximally, irrigated, and grafted with 40 mL of allograft bone. An HXLPE liner compatible with the implant's locking mechanism was not available, so a 28-mm internal diameter, 10-Mrad HXLPE liner was scored on the back surface using a high-speed burr and cemented into the shell.[39] A cobalt-chrome ball of the same neck length was implanted, resulting in equal limb lengths and good intraoperative stability. The patient was made weight bearing as tolerated and discharged 48 hours postoperatively. She underwent 6 weeks of physical therapy for gait training, abductor strengthening, and dislocation precaution education. At 1 year postoperatively, the patient had a Harris hip score of 98 and the graft appeared to be consolidating on radiographs (**Figure 5**).

CASE 2: FAILED CEMENTED THA

History

A 60-year-old woman presented with new-onset right hip pain 21 years after THA performed for hip dysplasia and secondary osteoarthritis. The patient reported shortening of the extremity over the last 2 years, a progressive limp, pain, and decreased ambulatory capacity (Harris hip score, 49; UCLA score, 4). Prior surgical notes indicated that the primary arthroplasty was performed via a transtrochanteric approach and used a cemented monoblock femoral component with a 22-mm femoral head and a cemented, all-polyethylene acetabular component; the acetabular reconstruction was augmented with native femoral head bulk allograft. The hip had not been evaluated in more than 15 years.[29-31]

Current Problem

A complete history was taken, and a thorough physical examination was performed. Radiographs (including an AP pelvis, Judet views, AP and lateral views of the hip, and a cross-table lateral) showed eccentric polyethylene wear, definite radiographic loosening of the acetabular component, and expansile osteolysis of the pelvis. The cemented monoblock femoral component is stably fixed and the trochanteric osteotomy had healed (**Figure 6**). The patient was instructed to curtail her activities, and revision surgery was planned.

Discussion

Evaluating this case may seem complex at first, but the basic tenets and tools outlined in Case 1 are very useful in simplifying this case. The patient underwent complex all-cemented THA with conventional polyethylene at a young age.[5] Several factors can be identified that might predispose this reconstruction to failure: patient factor (age), implant type (conventional polyethylene), and surgical technique (cement in young age and bulk graft supporting large portion of acetabular component).[5-7,13,14] Patient evaluation is straightforward in that the patient presented with pain, limp, and shortening, all clinical symptoms of implant loosening. The radiographs clearly indicate acetabular implant loosening and migration.

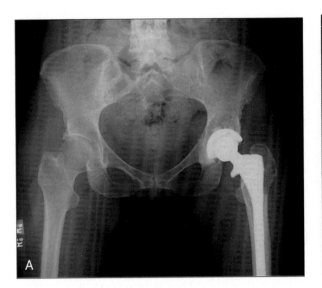
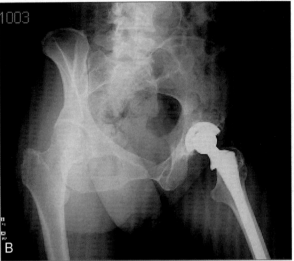

Figure 5 Postoperative radiographs of the patient described in Case 1. **A,** AP pelvic radiograph obtained 1 year postoperatively depicting consolidating periacetabular graft, centralized femoral head within new bearing, and a stable retained acetabular shell. **B,** Iliac oblique postoperative radiograph obtained 1 year postoperatively depicting consolidating particulate bone graft in posterior column and weight-bearing dome.

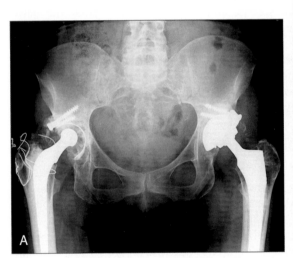
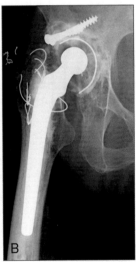
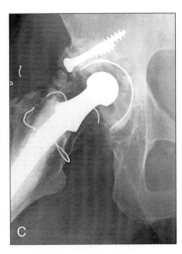

Figure 6   Radiographs of the 60-year-old woman described in Case 2. **A,** AP pelvic radiograph depicting eccentric wear, bulk allograft resorption, and loosened cemented acetabular component 21 years after cemented THA for dysplasia-related degeneration. **B,** Oblique pelvic radiograph depicting posterosuperior migration pattern of loosened acetabular component with associated bone loss. **C,** Lateral hip radiograph depicting well-fixed femoral component with stable cement mantle and 22-mm monoblock femoral head.

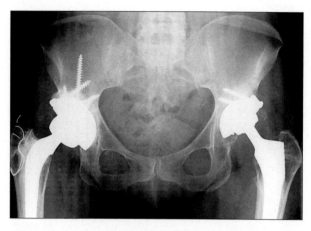

Figure 7 AP pelvic radiograph of the patient described in Case 2 depicting hip reconstruction 1 year postoperatively. Acetabular bone loss has been managed with metallic augments and the hip center restored. The bearing has been modified from a fixed 22-mm femoral head to a 40-mm bipolar.

Although not a metal-backed acetabular shell, it can be considered a type III acetabulum because it is loose and therefore needs to be revised (**see Table 1**).[35,36] The challenge is to create a stable construct. Metallic augments were chosen to manage bone loss and restore the hip center (medialization and proper orientation).[40,41] The bearing was modified to an HXLPE with a large femoral head via conversion of the monoblock 22-mm head to a 40-mm bipolar (a so-called tripolar construct).[15,16,42]

CASE MANAGEMENT AND OUTCOME

The patient underwent acetabular revision with femoral component retention using the tap-out tap-in technique.[43] Metallic pelvic augmentation allowed for restoration of hip center and management of posterosuperior bone loss (**Figure 4**).[40,41] The femoral bearing was modified to a 40-mm bipolar to enhance femoral offset and head-neck ratio.[42]

At 2-year follow-up, the patient had a Harris hip score of 92 and a UCLA score of 7. Radiographically, the acetabular components appeared to be stable with continued stability of the femoral component (**Figure 7**).

CASE 3: FAILED UNCEMENTED THA
History

A 75-year-old woman presented with a several-year history of progressive right hip pain 19 years after a THA. The patient reported increasing limp and decreased ambulatory capacity (Harris hip score, 52; UCLA score, 5). Prior surgical notes were unavailable. The hip had not been evaluated since the immediate postoperative period.[29-31]

Current Problem

A complete history revealed that the patient worked as a migrant field worker until 2 years prior to presentation.[5-7] Physical examination was remarkable for limb shortening, antalgic gait, painful range of motion, intact abductors, and a long posterior incision. Radiographs (AP pelvis and Judet views) showed eccentric polyethylene wear, a loosened and migrated cementless acetabular component with broken screws, and expansile osteolysis of the pelvis (**Figure 8, A through C**). Radiographs (AP and lateral views of the hip) indicated femoral component loosening and lysis with varus femoral remodeling and pedestal formation (**Figure 8, D and E**). The patient was instructed to curtail her activities, and revision surgery was planned.

Discussion

The basic tenets and tools outlined in the first case again are very useful in understanding this case. This patient underwent cementless THA with a conventional polyethylene bearing at age 56 with a very high activity level (UCLA score, 10).[5-7,13,14] Inspection of the radiographs identified an APR implant (Intermedics Orthopedics, Austin, TX). The APR was designed with patch porous coating on both the femoral and acetabular components.[10,11] Factors that could predispose to failure include patient factors (age, activity) and implant type (conventional polyethylene, patch porous cementless implants).[5-7,9,10,13,14] In this case, as in the prior two cases, the magnitude of failure at presentation is also likely related to a lack of postoperative follow-up.[29-31] Patient evaluation is straight-

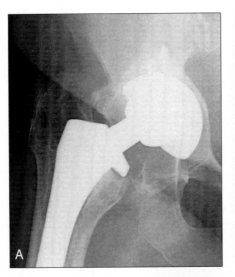
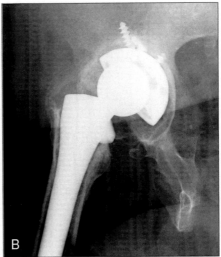
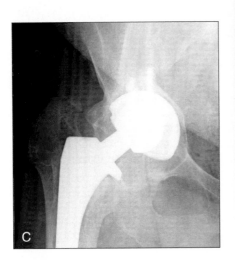
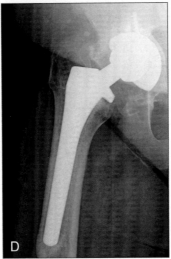
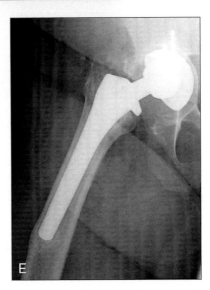

Figure 8 Radiographs of the 75-year-old woman described in Case 3. **A,** AP hip radiograph depicting eccentric wear, expansile acetabular lysis with acetabular component loosening, and broken screws. **B,** Iliac oblique pelvic radiograph depicting posterosuperior migration pattern of loosened acetabular component with associated bone loss. **C,** Obturator oblique pelvic radiograph depicting proximal migration and expansile lysis of anterior column. **D,** AP hip radiograph depicting previous acetabular findings as well as loosening of the femoral component with varus remodeling of femur and pedestal formation. Note divergent radiolucent lines (proximal lateral and inferior medial) and calcar reactive sclerosis consistent with loosening and varus migration. **E,** Lateral hip radiograph again depicting circumferential loosening and migration of femoral component and femoral remodeling.

forward: the patient presented with pain, limp, and shortening, all clinical symptoms of implant loosening. The radiographs indicate both acetabular and femoral implant loosening. The acetabular shell is considered a type III acetabulum because it is loose and therefore needs to be revised.[35,36] The femur had remodeled into varus secondary to loosening, creating a challenge for fixation.

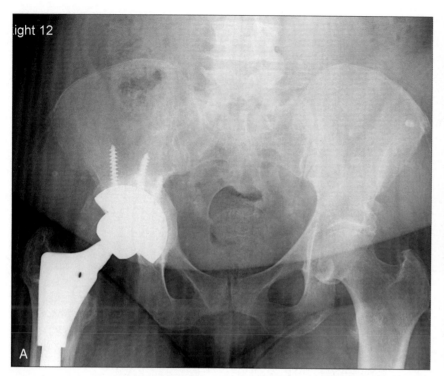
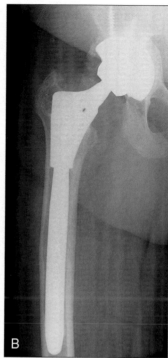

Figure 9 Postoperative radiographs of the patient described in Case 3. **A,** AP pelvic radiograph obtained 3 years postoperatively, depicting hip center restoration with large hemispherical acetabular component fixed with screws and lateralized by particulate grafting of expansile lysis. Note remodeling and incorporation of medial acetabular bone graft. Reconstructed offset is slightly greater than native state (contralateral side), contributing to the elimination of impingement and optimization of stability. **B,** AP hip radiograph depicting modular femoral component with proximal and distal fixation. Modularity allows independent sizing and fit of metaphysis and diaphysis.

CASE MANAGEMENT AND OUTCOME

The patient underwent acetabular and femoral revision with cementless components. The hip center was restored (lateralized) via particulate allograft in cavitary osteolytic defects and reconstructed with a cementless hemispherical shell with additional screws (**Figure 9, A**).[35,36] The new bearing choice was a 10-Mrad HXLPE articulating with a cobalt chrome head.[15,16] After removal of the pedestal, the varus femoral deformity was reconstructed with a cementless modular implant, that allowed independent sizing of the metaphysis and diaphysis (**Figure 9, B**). Fixation of the femoral component was achieved in the metaphysis as well as the diaphysis distal to the removed pedestal (**Figure 9**). Stability of the construct was optimized by choosing a femoral implant with increased offset and a 36-mm bearing.

At 4-year follow-up, the patient had a Harris hip score of 98 and a UCLA score of 7. Radiographs confirmed both acetabular and femoral component osseous stability.

STRATEGIES TO MINIMIZE COMMON COMPLICATIONS

Strategies to minimize osteolysis fall under the categories of early detection, prevention, and treatment.

Early Detection

Routine follow-up including radiographs is the mainstay of early detection.

Prevention

Strategies for osteolysis prevention include appropriate patient selection, proper surgical technique, and the development and use of more wear-resistant bearing surfaces.

Treatment

In the young patient, medical management of hip pain should be extended as long as possible and nonarthroplasty surgical options should be considered. When performing an arthroplasty, the surgeon should always attempt to minimize the joint reactive force and bearing stress by medializing the acetabular component, preventing acetabular abduction greater than 55°, and restoring femoral offset. In patients at high risk for bearing wear and subsequent osteolysis, the use of newer, low-wear bearings should be considered. Current metal-on-metal, ceramic-on-ceramic, and HXLPE bearings all have displayed improved wear characteristics in vitro. The hope is that THAs performed with modern bearings will not be subject to the rates of osteolysis and late failure observed with conventional polyethylene bearings. It should be noted, however, that each modern bearing couple has its unique shortcomings and may be subject to unknown modes of late failure. Continued close observation in well-controlled clinical studies is necessary to determine the long-term outcome of THA performed with modern bearings. In the future, medical management of periprosthetic bone loss may be effective. At present, however, revision surgery is the mainstay of osteolysis treatment and should be timed, when possible, to minimize complexity by allowing prosthetic retention and bearing exchange.

REFERENCES

1. Archibeck MJ, Jacobs JJ, Roebuck KA, Glant TT: The basic science of periprosthetic osteolysis. *Instr Course Lect* 2001;50:185-195.

2. Saleh KJ, Thongtrangan I, Schwarz EM: Osteolysis: Medical and surgical approaches. *Clin Orthop Relat Res* 2004;427:138-147.

3. Oparaugo PC, Clarke IC, Malchau H, Herberts P: Correlation of wear debris-induced osteolysis and revision with volumetric wear-rates of polyethylene: A survey of 8 reports in the literature. *Acta Orthop Scand* 2001;72:22-28.

4. Jacobs JJ, Goodman SB, Sumner DR, Hallab NJ: Biologic response to orthopaedic implants, in Buckwalter JA, Einhorn TA, Simon SR (eds): *Orthopaedic Basic Science*, ed 2. Rosemont, IL, American Academy of Orthopaedic Surgeons, 2000, pp 401-426.

5. Nercessian OA, Joshi RP, Martin G, Su BW, Eftekhar NS: Influence of demographic and technical variables on the incidence of osteolysis in Charnley primary low friction hip arthroplasty. *J Arthroplasty* 2003;18:631-637.

6. Joshi RP, Eftekhar NS, McMahon DJ, Nercessian OA: Osteolysis after Charnley primary low-friction arthroplasty: A comparison of two matched paired groups. *J Bone Joint Surg Br* 1998;80:585-590.

7. McClung CD, Zahiri CA, Higa JK, Amstutz HC, Schmalzried TP: Relationship between body mass index and activity in hip or knee arthroplasty patients. *J Orthop Res* 2000;18:35-39.

8. Dowd JE, Sychterz CJ, Young AM, Engh CA: Characterization of long-term femoral-head-penetration rates: Association with and prediction of osteolysis. *J Bone Joint Surg Am* 2000;82:1102-1107.

9. Thanner J, Karrholm J, Malchau H, Herberts P: Poor outcome of the PCA and Harris-Galante hip prostheses: Randomized study of 171 arthroplasties with 9-year follow-up. *Acta Orthop Scand* 1999;70:155-162.

10. Martell JM, Pierson RH, Jacobs JJ, Rosenberg AG, Maley M, Galante JO: Primary total hip reconstruction with a titanium fiber-coated prosthesis inserted without cement. *J Bone Joint Surg Am* 1993;75:554-571.

11. Schmalzried TP, Jasty M, Harris WH: Periprosthetic bone loss in total hip arthroplasty: Polyethylene wear debris and the concept of the effective joint space. *J Bone Joint Surg Am* 1992;74:849-863.

12. Patil S, Bergula A, Chen PC, Colwell CW, D'Lima DD: Polyethylene wear and acetabular component orientation. *J Bone Joint Surg Am* 2003;85(Suppl 4):56-63.

13. Lee PC, Shih CH, Chen WJ, Tu YK, Tai CL: Early polyethylene wear and osteolysis in cementless total hip arthroplasty: The influence of femoral head size and polyethylene thickness. *J Arthroplasty* 1999;14:976-981.

14. Orishimo KF, Claus AM, Sychterz CJ, Engh CA: Relationship between polyethylene wear and osteolysis in hips with a second-generation porous-coated cementless cup after seven years of follow-up. *J Bone Joint Surg Am* 2003;85:1095-1099.

15. Muratoglu OK, O'Connor DO, Bragdon CR, et al: Gradient crosslinking of UHMWPE using irradiation in molten state for total joint arthroplasty. *Biomaterials* 2002;23:717-724.

16. Manning DW, Chiang PP, Martell JM, Galante JO, Harris WH: In vivo comparative wear study of traditional and highly cross-linked polyethylene in total hip arthroplasty. *J Arthroplasty* 2005;20:880-886.

17. Capello WN, Dantonio JA, Feinberg JR, Manley MT: Alternative bearing surfaces: Alumina ceramic bearings for total hip arthroplasty. *Instr Course Lect* 2005;54:171-176.

18. Sedel L, Nizard R, Bizot P, Meunier A: Perspective of a 20-year experience with ceramic-on-ceramic articulation in total hip replacement. *Semin Arthroplasty* 1998;9:123-134.

19. Walter WL, O'Toole GC, Walter WK, Ellis A, Zicat BA: Squeaking in ceramic-on-ceramic hips: The importance of acetabular component orientation. *J Arthroplasty* 2007;22:496-503. Epub 2007 Mar 28.

20. Cuckler JM: The rationale for metal-on-metal total hip arthroplasty. *Clin Orthop Relat Res* 2005;441:132-136.

21. Brown SR, Davies WA, DeHeer DH, Swanson AB: Long-term survival of McKee-Farrar total hip prostheses. *Clin Orthop Relat Res* 2002;402:157-163.

22. Jacobsson SA, Djerf K, Wahlstrom O: Twenty-year results of McKee-Farrar versus Charnley prosthesis. *Clin Orthop Relat Res* 1996;329(Suppl):S60-S68.

23. Urban RM, Tomlinson MJ, Hall DJ, Jacobs JJ: Accumulation in liver and spleen of metal particles generated at nonbearing surfaces in hip arthroplasty. *J Arthroplasty* 2004;19(8, Suppl 3)94-101.

24. Visuri T, Pukkala E, Paavolainen P, Pulkkinen P, Riska EB: Cancer risk after metal on metal and polyethylene on metal total hip arthroplasty. *Clin Orthop Relat Res* 1996;329(Suppl):S280-S289.

25. Masse A, Bosetti M, Buratti C, et al: Ion release and chromosomal damage from total hip prostheses with metal-on-metal articulation. *J Biomed Mater Res B Appl Biomater* 2003;67:750-757.

26. Hallab NJ, Anderson S, Caicedo M, et al: Immune responses correlate with serum-metal in metal-on-metal hip arthroplasty. *J Arthroplasty* 2004;19(Suppl 3):88-93.

27. Davies AP, Willert HG, Campbell PA, et al: An unusual lymphocytic perivascular infiltration in tissues around contemporary metal-on-metal joint replacements. *J Bone Joint Surg Am* 2005;87:18-27.

28. Milosev I, Trebse R, Kovac S, Cör A, Pisot V: Survivorship and retrieval analysis of Sikomet metal-on-metal total hip replacements at a mean of seven years. *J Bone Joint Surg Am* 2006;88:1173-1182.

29. Berry DJ: Management of osteolysis around total hip arthroplasty. *Orthopedics* 1999;22:805-808.

30. NIH consensus conference: Total hip replacement. NIH Consensus Development Panel on Total Hip Replacement. *JAMA* 1995;273:1950-1956.

31. Teeny SM, York SC, Mesko JW, Rea RE: Long-term follow-up care recommendations after total hip and knee arthroplasty: Results of the American Association of Hip and Knee Surgeons' member survey. *J Arthroplasty* 2003;18:954-962.

32. Talmo CT, Shanbhag AS, Rubash HE: Nonsurgical management of osteolysis: Challenges and opportunities. *Clin Orthop Relat Res* 2006;453:254-264.

33. Arabmotlagh M, Pilz M, Warzecha J: Changes of femoral periprosthetic bone mineral density 6 years after treatment with alendronate following total hip arthroplasty. *J Orthop Res* 2008 Aug 27. Epub ahead of print.

34. Rubash HE, Dorr LD, Jacobs JJ, et al: Does alendronate inhibit the progression of periprosthetic osteolysis? *Trans Orthop Res Soc* 2004;29:1888.

35. Maloney WJ, Paprosky W, Engh CA, Rubash H: Surgical treatment of pelvic osteolysis. *Clin Orthop Relat Res* 2001;393:78-84.

36. Rubash HE, Sinha RK, Paprosky W, Engh CA, Maloney WJ: A new classification system for the management of acetabular osteolysis after total hip arthroplasty. *Instr Course Lect* 1999;48:37-42.

37. Boucher HR, Lynch C, Young AM, Engh CA Jr, Engh C Sr: Dislocation after polyethylene liner exchange in total hip arthroplasty. *J Arthroplasty* 2003;18:654-657.

38. Manning D, Chaing P, Martell J: In vivo comparative wear study of traditional and highly cross-linked polyethylene in total hip arthroplasty. *J Arthroplasty* 2005;20:880-886.

39. Yoon TR, Seon JK, Song EK: Cementation of a metal-inlay polyethylene liner into a stable metal shell in revision total hip arthroplasty. *J Arthroplasty* 2005;20:652-657.

40. Paprosky WG, Sporer SS, Murphy
    BP: Addressing severe bone defi-
    ciency: What a cage will not do.
    J Arthroplasty 2007;22(4 Suppl
    1):111-115.

41. Sporer SS, Paprosky WG: The use
    of a trabecular metal acetabular
    component and trabecular metal
    augment for severe acetabular
    defects. *J Arthroplasty* 2006;
    21(6 Suppl 2):83-86.

42. Guyen O, Chen QS:
    Unconstrained tripolar hip
    implants: Effect on hip stability.
    Clin Orthop Relat Res 2007;455:
    202-208.

43. Nabors ED, Liebelt R, Mattingly
    DA, Bierbaum BE: Removal and
    reinsertion of cemented femoral
    components during acetabular
    revision. *J Arthroplasty*
    1996;11:146-52.

Chapter 8

EVALUATION OF THE PAINFUL TOTAL HIP ARTHROPLASTY

Brett Levine, MD, MS
Kevin J. Bozic, MD, MBA
*Michael D. Ries, MD
*Thomas Parker Vail, MD

CASE PRESENTATION

A 64-year-old man who had undergone cementless total hip arthroplasty (THA) 4 years previously presented with posterolateral hip and thigh pain. He also had a history of chronic low back pain treated with long-term narcotic medications. Pain developed immediately after surgery without a significant period of relief. His symptoms were localized primarily to the thigh and, to a lesser extent, were referred to the buttock region. At presentation, the patient reported persistent pain that was aggravated with weight-bearing activities.

The patient ambulated with a mild Trendelenburg gait. Passive hip motion was 0° to 100° of flexion, 10° of internal rotation, 30° of external rotation, 30° of abduction, and 20° of adduction. Combined hip flexion and internal rotation was associated with moderate thigh pain. Mild tenderness on palpation was present over the greater trochanter and low back. Radiographs showed evidence of an osseointegrated cylindrical canal-filling femoral stem and a well-fixed acetabular component (**Figure 1**). Routine workup for infection and other sources of pain was negative. The pain was ultimately attributed to stress transfer at the stem tip.

DISCUSSION
Recognizing the Problem and High-Risk Situations

Despite a high level of reported success after THA, it is not uncommon for patients to present with pain in the surgical hip at some point during follow-up.[1] With a continued increase in the number of THAs being performed annually (572,000 projected by 2030), a steady rise can be expected in the number of patients who present with pain after THA.[2] Identifying the source of pain in these patients is often very difficult and may lead to frustration on the part of

*Michael D. Ries, MD, or the department with which he is affiliated has received royalties from Smith & Nephew. Thomas Parker Vail, MD, or the department with which he is affiliated has received research or institutional support from Zimmer, has received royalties from DePuy, and is a consultant for or an employee of DePuy.

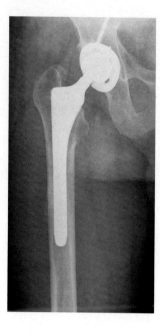

Figure 1 AP radiograph obtained 4 years after cementless THA in a 64-year-old man with persistent thigh pain demonstrates a well-fixed cylindrical, diaphyseal-engaging stem.

TABLE 1 Differential Diagnosis of the Painful THA

Extrinsic causes

Hernia (femoral, inguinal, obturator)
Intra-abdominal or genitourinary pathology
Lumbar spine disease
Disk herniation (radiculopathy)
Spondylolysis/spondylolisthesis
Stenosis (neurogenic claudication)
Malignancy/metastases
Metabolic bone disease (Paget disease, osteomalacia)
Nerve injury/irritation (femoral, meralgia paresthetica, sciatic)
Neuropathy (eg, diabetic)
Peripheral vascular disease

Intrinsic causes

End of stem pain (modulus mismatch)
Infection
Inflammatory bursitis/tendinitis (iliopsoas, trochanteric)
Mechanical loosening of acetabular or femoral component
Occult instability
Osteolysis and synovitis secondary to polyethylene wear
Periprosthetic fracture
Stress fracture (pubic rami)
Trochanteric nonunion

the surgeon and the patient. Algorithms have been suggested to guide surgeons in obtaining the appropriate tests and imaging studies for a complete diagnostic workup of a painful THA.[3] Even with such algorithms, accurately distinguishing the source of pain remains a challenging task.

The overall differential diagnosis of a painful THA comprises a daunting list of potential causes (**Table 1**). To simplify this process, Bozic and Rubash[3] classified the sources of a painful THA as either intrinsic or extrinsic to the hip joint.

Intrinsic Causes of Pain

Pain associated with a pathologic process within or adjacent to the hip joint is called an intrinsic cause of pain. The most common forms of intrinsic pain include inflammatory muscle/tendon/bursal conditions, periprosthetic joint infection, mechanical loosening, periprosthetic fracture, and occult instability.

Periprosthetic joint infection is a rare but potentially devastating cause of pain after THA. Because of the possibility of dire consequences, infection should always be considered and thoroughly investigated for during the diagnostic workup (see chapter 6). Mechanical loosening of the implant can occur early or late and is typically associated with start-up pain.

Osteolysis-associated inflammation and subtle instability or subluxation can also lead to a painful THA. Similarly, a mismatch in the modulus of elasticity between large, stiff, metallic implants and the bone can be associated with thigh pain.

Trochanteric bursitis and iliopsoas tendinitis are two common musculoskeletal conditions associated with THA. Numerous bursae surround the greater trochanter, and they can be related to lateral hip pain after THA, particularly when associated with an anterolateral exposure to the hip or an increase in femoral offset. Groin pain with resisted hip flexion is found in patients with inflammation of the iliopsoas tendon. This tendinopathy is occasionally associated with retroverted and oversized acetabular components (**Figure 2**), but it also can occur in the presence of well-placed and appropriately sized implants.

Less common intrinsic sources of pain include stress fracture, atraumatic periprosthetic fracture, nonunion, and heterotopic ossification. Stress fractures can be seen in the pubic rami (**Figure 3**) and are more common in women and in patients with osteopenia. These fractures typically occur during the first postoperative year and present as acute onset groin pain. Atraumatic periprosthetic fractures may affect the greater trochanter when associated with osteolysis or severe stress shielding of the proximal femur. If a transtrochanteric approach is used for exposure, nonunion (range, 1% to 38%) of the greater trochanter or soft-tissue irritation adjacent to the hardware used for fixation can be a source of continued pain.[4] Heterotopic ossification after THA is more often associated with limited hip motion, but occasionally it can contribute to pain. Neurogenic pain is more common after knee surgery or trauma than hip surgery, but it also can serve as a pain generator after THA.

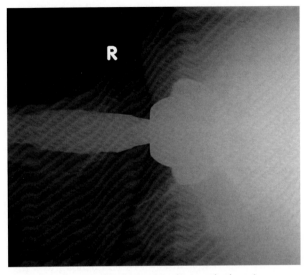

Figure 2 Cross-table lateral radiograph showing a slightly retroverted acetabular component that caused iliopsoas tendinitis.

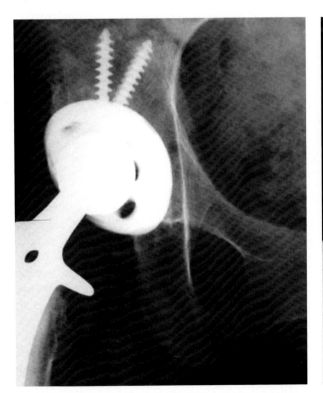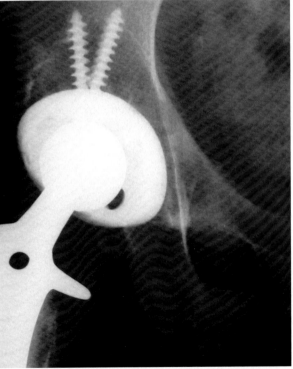

Figure 3 Radiographs of a patient who reported several months of ipsilateral groin pain starting approximately 8 months following THA. **A,** AP radiograph taken 6 weeks postoperatively. **B,** Repeat radiograph obtained at 12 months postoperatively shows evidence of a healed stress fracture of the superior pubic ramus.

Extrinsic Causes of Pain

Sources of pain located outside the hip are described as extrinsic causes of pain after THA. These are most commonly related to lumbar spine disease, peripheral vascular disease, and referred pain. Spinal stenosis, disk herniation, spondylolysis, and spondylolisthesis can all be coupled with perceived hip pain and should be ruled out as a source of pain before and after THA.[5] Vascular claudication of the aorto-iliac system and nerve injury/irritation (sciatic, femoral, meralgia paresthetica) can cause groin, buttock or thigh pain after THA. Hernia (femoral, inguinal, obturator) and genitourinary pathology also may refer pain to the hip region from the abdominal and pelvic cavities, respectively. Complex regional pain syndrome, metabolic diseases (Paget disease, osteomalacia), and primary or metastatic bone cancers are less frequent extrinsic causes of pain after THA.[3]

Evaluating the Problem

A plethora of diagnostic tests can be useful in the evaluation of a painful THA. Before ordering ancillary tests, however, a thorough history and physical examination should be conducted because this can narrow the differential diagnosis and help the physician avoid ordering unnecessary tests. Haphazardly ordering diagnostic tests is inefficient and not cost-effective, and it may even hinder the process of reaching a definitive diagnosis.

History

A detailed medical history should be obtained, including pertinent clinical symptoms, past medical history, and past surgical history (including surgical reports and office notes related to prior surgeries). The evaluation should include an accurate description of the character, location, onset, and severity of the pain as well as exacerbating and/or alleviating factors. This thorough evaluation of the pain symptoms can lead to a more focused diagnostic workup and is a crucial element of the history. **Table 2** lists various types of pain commonly reported after THA and their typical causes.

A detailed history also includes a review of previous surgical reports, especially noting any perioperative complications that may have occurred during the index procedure. A history of prolonged wound drainage or delayed wound healing requiring postoperative antibiotics or frequent dressing changes increases the likelihood of a chronic infection. Episodes of instability or a return to the operating room is also an important clue to the etiology of the pain. Acute onset hip pain after an invasive (eg, dental or gastrointestinal) procedure, following a systemic illness, or coincident with a distant site infection raises the suspicion of hematogenous seeding of the THA.

Obtaining a complete past medical history also is important. Diabetes mellitus, psoriatic arthritis, rheumatoid arthritis, obesity, immunosuppression, poor nutrition, renal failure/dialysis, and skin disorders are conditions associated with an increased risk for infection after THA.[3]

Physical Examination

A complete musculoskeletal physical examination should be performed with a focus on the hip, adjacent joints, and low back. The patient should be gowned and should have shoes and socks removed to allow inspection and palpation of the lower extremities and back. In general, physical examination begins with inspection of the skin, including the surgical incision, potential areas for decubitus ulcers (sacrum and heels), and the foot and ankle region, for evidence of venous stasis and circulatory status. The surgical site should be evaluated for erythema, fluctuance, calor, drainage, and sinus tracts; the location of the incision also should be noted, as it can provide evidence as to the direction of the prior surgical approach. Comparison with the contralateral limb is helpful in assessing muscle wasting and evidence of disuse atrophy. Palpation should be performed concomitantly with inspection of the lower extremities. Fluctuant masses, expressible drainage, and trochanteric bursitis may be elicited during this part of the examination. Estimated leg lengths can be observed by palpating the medial malleoli; true (anterior superior iliac spine to the medial malleolus) and apparent (umbilicus to the medial malleolus) leg lengths can be confirmed using a tape measure. If serial measurements show shortening of the lower extremity, mechanical loosening of the implant should be suspected. Palpation of the groin area can assess for an inguinal hernia or pubic rami stress fractures.

TABLE 2 Types of Pain Reported After THA and Typical Causes

Type of Pain	Typical Causes
Early, persistent	Prosthetic infection Periprosthetic fracture Misdiagnosis of original condition causing the pain Mechanical complication of prosthesis
Late, arising after a period of good function[3]	Aseptic loosening Late infection Periprosthetic stress fracture Wear-related osteolysis
Thigh pain	Conditions surrounding the femoral stem/femur
Lateral hip pain	Trochanteric bursitis
Groin pain	Conditions relating to acetabular component
Start-up pain that improves with activity	Implant loosening/micromotion
Start-up thigh pain in patient with cementless, diaphyseal-engaging stem	Stress transfer (modulus of elasticity mismatch) from stem tip to femoral diaphysis Implant micromotion
Severe pain with activity that improves significantly with rest	Periprosthetic fracture Loose implant Vascular claudication Neurogenic condition
Unrelenting or night pain	Deep infection Synovial irritation secondary to wear particles Malignancy
Radicular pain Dysesthesias radiating from buttocks to below the knee	Neurogenic; related to lumbar spine disorders such as disk herniation, spinal stenosis, spondylolisthesis

Range of motion at the hip, knee, and ankle is then evaluated for asymmetry. Pain and limitations in passive motion may signify an intrinsic source of pain or impingement. Similarly, provocative movements for anterior and/or posterior dislocation may elicit apprehension by the patient typical of instability. On the other hand, pain with active range of motion of the hip, particularly at the extremes, may indicate implant loosening. Iliopsoas tendinitis is classically diagnosed when examination reveals pain on resisted flexion or passive extension of the hip.[6]

A complete neurologic evaluation is then performed, including reflex testing, motor and sensory function testing, the straight-leg raise test, Babinski signs, and testing for lower extremity clonus. Peripheral nerve injuries involving the femoral nerve (quadriceps weakness) and sciatic nerve (foot drop) can be diagnosed during a thorough neurologic examination. Nerve irritation, lumbar spine pathology, and peripheral nerve injury should be readily detected and ruled out as a source of pain after THA. The patient's gait can then be assessed for antalgia or a Trendelenburg gait. Close observation of the gait pattern can reveal important information regarding the underlying etiology of the patient's pain.

Laboratory Workup

Appropriate serologic testing should be ordered for all patients with a painful THA, particularly if the history and physical examination raise the suspicion for deep infection. The erythrocyte sedimentation rate (ESR) and C-reactive protein (CRP) level are the inflammatory markers most commonly obtained to screen for prosthetic joint infection. A white blood cell (WBC) count, although often ordered, has been shown repeatedly to be highly inaccurate in diagnosing periprosthetic joint infections.[7,8] Schinsky and associates[8] found no infections when both the ESR and CRP were normal and the history and physical examination were not suspicious for infection. Similar reports have confirmed that an ESR and CRP combined with a thorough history and physical examination comprise an accurate screening tool for the diagnosis of periprosthetic joint infection.

Several conditions may artificially elevate the ESR and CRP level, however, so the specificity of these tests in patients with these conditions is much lower than in patients without these confounding comorbidities. Chronic inflammatory conditions such as rheumatoid arthritis or lupus erythematosus, systemic illness, recent surgical intervention, and pregnancy are just a few of the conditions that may elevate these nonspecific markers of inflammation. Typically, the CRP level returns to normal values within 3 to 6 weeks after surgery and the ESR by 6 months. Occasionally, however, the ESR remains elevated for up to 1 year after an uncomplicated THA. In the absence of these confounding conditions, an elevated ESR and CRP level in the setting of a painful THA is suggestive of infection and can be evaluated further with a hip aspiration (including synovial fluid WBC count with differential and culture).

Most recently, Di Cesare and associates[7] and Bottner and associates[10] have reported on the use of interleukin-6 (IL-6) levels in the diagnosis of prosthetic joint infections. Di Cesare and associates[7] found the following characteristics for the IL-6 test: sensitivity, 100%; specificity, 95%; positive predictive value, 89%; negative predictive value, 100%; and accuracy, 97%. This test, however, is costly and

is not widely available, so the clinical utility and cost effectiveness of IL-6 as a diagnostic tool for patients with suspected periprosthetic joint infections remains unproved at this time.

Radiographic Evaluation

Patients with a painful THA should have a complete series of plain radiographs (AP hip, frog-lateral, shoot-through lateral, and AP pelvis) taken when they present, and all available prior radiographs and studies should be reviewed for comparison. A series of radiographs taken at a single office visit is often insufficient and is much less powerful as a diagnostic tool than serial radiographs, including preoperative, immediate postoperative, and latest follow-up. When comparing these serial radiographs for perceived interval changes, however, it is important to consider variations in technique such as penetration, magnification, patient orientation, weight-bearing versus non–weight-bearing, and rotation of the lower extremities.

Criteria for radiographic loosening of cemented and cementless femoral and acetabular components have been well established.[11-14] Harris and McGann[12] categorized radiographic loosening of cemented femoral components as definite loosening (implant migration, fracture of stem or the cement mantle), probable loosening (continuous or >2 mm radiolucent line at the bone-cement interface), and possible loosening (50% to 100% radiolucent line at the bone-cement interface). Engh and associates[11] reported on radiographic signs of osseointegration of porous femoral components, describing major and minor signs of bony ingrowth. Major signs of osseointegration include the absence of reactive, sclerotic lines around the porous coating of the implant and evidence of endosteal spot welds (typically found at the junction of the coated and noncoated areas of the implant). Minor signs of bony ingrowth are calcar atrophy, proximal stress shielding, a stable distal stem, and the absence of a pedestal. Progressive implant subsidence and the presence of circumferential sclerotic lines around the component signify failure of osseointegration and loosening.

Criteria for radiographic signs of loosening of cemented acetabular components have been described by the Hodgkinson classification.[15] This system defines 4 types of radiographic demarcation of the cup: type 0—no demarcation; type 1—demarcation of the outer one third, type 2—demarcation of outer and middle thirds; type 3—complete demarcation; type 4—socket migration. More recently, Hartofilakidis and associates[16] defined acetabular implant loosening as migration of more than 2 mm in any direction or the presence of a continuous radiolucent line of more than 1 mm at the cement-bone interface. Yoder and associates[14] described the criteria for loosening of a cementless acetabular component as migration of the implant greater than 4 mm, change in abduction angle greater than 4°, or development of a radiolucent line greater than 2 mm around in all three radiographic zones around the cup (as described by DeLee and Charnley[17]). The presence of broken screws (fatigue fracture) also signifies micromotion and failure of osseointegration of the acetabular component. In addition, Udomkiat and associates[13] found that progressive radiolucent lines of at least 1 mm thickness appearing after the second year and a radiolucent line greater than 2 mm in any zone were indicators of cementless acetabular component loosening.

Close scrutiny of the plain radiographs for osteolysis in the form of radiolucent lines and expansile osteolytic lesions is necessary and should be documented in the appropriate zones in both the femur and acetabulum. Progressive lucencies or large expansile lesions may be implicated directly as a source of pain (fracture, implant loosening) or can indicate significant wear-associated synovitis. Subtle signs of periprosthetic joint infection also may be present and should be looked for carefully. These include periosteal new bone formation, generalized osteolysis, endosteal scalloping, and rapid bony destruction.

Aspiration, Injection, and Arthroscopy

Preoperative arthrocentesis of the hip under fluoroscopic guidance for diagnosing infection has been reported to have a variable sensitivity, ranging from 50% to 93%.[18] Recent studies, however, have reported improved success rates (sensitivity and specificity of 82% and 91%, respectively) when appropriate criteria are used to select patients for this test.[8,18] Recommended indications for preoperative aspiration include presence of one or more of the following: (1) radiographic or clinical suspicion of prosthetic joint infection; (2) elevated ESR and/or CRP level; (3) medical conditions that may falsely elevate the ESR/CRP values, making them unreliable; (4) history of wound infection or healing problems; and (5) implant failure within the first 5 years after THA.[18] Aspiration should be performed in the operating room or fluoroscopy suite under sterile conditions. Tissue biopsy has not been proved to increase the accuracy of diagnosis during aspiration and is not currently recommended.[18,19] Fluid obtained during aspiration should be sent for synovial fluid WBC count with differential as well as aerobic, anaerobic, fungal, and acid-fast bacilli cultures. Two concerns regarding hip aspiration after THA are the possible introduction of a bacterial contaminant to the hip and the possibility of unintentionally contaminating the specimen.

The synovial fluid cell count has been shown to be a reliable test for diagnosing periprosthetic joint infection, particularly when evaluated in conjunction with the ESR and CRP level.[8,20,21] Schinsky and associates[8] recommend using the following values as the cut-off to establish infection of a THA: 3,000 WBC/mL when both the ESR and CRP are elevated, and 9,000 WBC/mL when either the ESR or CRP is elevated. For the first situation (>3,000 WBC/mL, ESR and CRP elevated), the following results were reported: sensitivity, 90%; specificity, 91%; positive predictive value, 95%; negative predictive value, 82%; and accuracy, 90%. This WBC level is strikingly lower than previous reports, in which infection was diagnosed at 25,000 to 80,000 WBC/mL.[9,22] As an adjunct to the cell count, Schinsky and associates[8] suggested using >80% polymorphonuclear cells to help confirm periprosthetic infection. Gram stain is currently not recommended because of its poor sensitivity.

Intra-articular injection of the hip with a local anesthetic can be helpful in defining the location of the pain as either intra- or extra-capsular. Patients typically experience transient relief of symptoms with such an injection if the pain generator is located within the hip capsule. Braunstein and associates[23] found that 91% of patients experienced complete relief within 20 minutes of an intra-articular injection of local anesthetic when the source of pain was intracapsular. Injection may be used similarly to diagnose pain suspected of originating in the lumbosacral spine, thereby ruling out THA as the source of pain.

The use of hip arthroscopy to evaluate and treat painful THAs was recently reviewed retrospectively by McCarthy and associates.[24] They reported on 14 patients (16 hips) who underwent arthroscopy after THA, 4 with a known diagnosis and 10 with persistent pain despite negative diagnostic studies. In 12 of the hips, arthroscopy led to a successful treatment or directed a treatment subsequently leading to a good outcome. No intraoperative complications were reported, and the group concluded that in select cases arthroscopy may play a role in diagnosing and treating patients with unexplained pain after THA.[24]

Nuclear Medicine Studies

Several different nuclear medicine studies can potentially be helpful in the evaluation of a painful THA, including technetium-99 labeled methylene diphosphonate (^{99}TcMDP) scans, indium 111(^{111}In)-labeled leukocyte scans, gallium citrate (^{67}Ga) scans, and combined technetium-99m sulfur colloid/^{111}indium-labeled leukocyte scans. ^{99}TcMDP scans are commonly used to investigate possible component loosening. Despite ^{99}TcMDP being a sensitive indicator of metabolically active bone, it is quite nonspecific, and increased uptake can be seen with loosening, infection, heterotopic ossification, stress fractures, modulus mismatch, tumors, metabolic bone disease, and complex regional pain syndrome.[25] A secondary concern with ^{99}TcMDP scans is the fact that increased uptake may be seen around an uncomplicated THA for up to 2 years after surgery.[26] The utility of ^{99}TcMDP scans is currently controversial: Lieberman and associates[27] found that ^{99}TcMDP bone scans were no more effective in elucidating a diagnosis than serial plain radiographs in their series of 54 hip revisions; Nagoya and associates[28] showed 88% sensitivity and 90% specificity when a three-phase ^{99}TcMDP scan was used for detecting periprosthetic infection. Despite this controversy, ^{99}TcMDP remains an option for evaluating a painful THA (**Figure 4**).

A ^{67}Ga scan in conjunction with a ^{99}TcMDP scan may help differentiate septic from aseptic loosening. Mixed results have been reported with this technique, and the test has largely been supplanted by ^{111}In

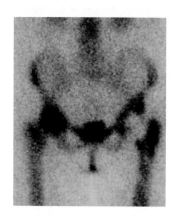

Figure 4 Three-phase bone scan showing increased uptake around the greater trochanter in a patient reporting lateral thigh pain after THA indicative of an occult periprosthetic fracture of the greater trochanter. There is also increased periacetabular uptake consistent with the plain radiograph findings of retroacetabular osteolysis.

leukocyte scintigraphy.[3] ^{111}In scans have a higher sensitivity and specificity for excluding periprosthetic joint infection than do ^{99}TcMDP and ^{67}Ga scans, either alone or in combination,[29] but Scher and associates[30] found that ^{111}In was only slightly better. They studied 143 hip and knee arthroplasties and found a positive predictive value of 54% and a negative predictive value of 95% using ^{111}In scintigraphy. Overall, this suggests that a negative scan is useful to exclude infection as the source for a painful total joint arthroplasty. Currently, combined technetium-99m sulfur colloid/^{111}indium-labeled leukocyte scanning is the preferred imaging modality for infected total joint arthroplasties.[31] This technique was developed to improve upon the high false-positive rate of ^{111}In scintigraphy, which occurs because physiologic marrow packing can cause the appearance of increased uptake in an otherwise normal scan.

FDG-PET is a new high-resolution imaging study that detects the energy consumption of tissues in three dimensions. Pill and associates[31] compared combined technetium-99m sulfur colloid/^{111}indium-labeled leukocyte scanning with FDG-PET in the diagnosis of periprosthetic infection. Results for FDG-PET scan in diagnosing infection were as follows: 95.2% sensitivity, 93% specificity, 80% positive predictive value, and a 98.5% negative predictive value. This compared with 50% sensitivity, 95.1% specificity, 41.7% positive predictive value, and

88.6% negative predictive value for the combined technetium-99m sulfur colloid/[111]indium-labeled leukocyte scan. Access to FDG-PET scans is currently available at a limited number of centers, however, and it remains a relatively expensive test.

Magnetic Resonance Imaging

Thanks to metal artifact–sparing techniques, MRI can now be used to obtain good quality images of the bone-implant interface and the surrounding soft tissues after THA.[32-34] This technique allows improved soft-tissue visualization after total joint arthroplasty without the ionizing radiation exposure of CT scans. Cooper and associates[32] reviewed a series of 21 hips in patients with persistent pain after THA and found that MRI was able to detect soft-tissue pathology in the periprosthetic tissues in all 21 cases. Consistent visualization of the bone-implant interface was demonstrated, and the following periprosthetic pathology was found: abductor tendinosis (17 cases), periacetabular osteolysis (10 cases), femoral osteolysis (7 cases), particle-induced synovitis (7 cases), iliopsoas bursitis/tendinosis (11 cases), trochanteric bursitis (2 cases), and soft-tissue ganglia (2 cases). Selective use of MRI with a modified pulse sequence may allow accurate diagnosis of unexplained pain that persists in a small percentage of patients after THA.

CASE MANAGEMENT

Treatment

In the 64-year-old man described initially, a course of nonsurgical therapy including nonsteroidal anti-inflammatory drugs, physical therapy, and activity modification was tried, but it failed to relieve the symptoms. Revision was performed using an extended trochanteric osteotomy (ETO) to extract the femoral component. A modular, tapered, cementless stem and allograft strut were used to reduce the distal inner stem diameter and increase diaphyseal bone rigidity (**Figure 5**).

Outcome

One year after the revision, the osteotomy and allograft had healed, but the patient continued to have

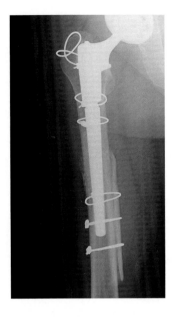

Figure 5 In the patient shown in Figure 1, revision THA was performed with a modular, tapered, cementless stem and allograft strut. AP radiograph obtained 1 year after revision demonstrates that the ETO and allograft have healed, yet the patient continued to have persistent pain similar to that before the revision surgery.

enigmatic pain similar to that which he experienced before revision THA. This case demonstrates a failure of revision surgery to effectively alleviate thigh pain after cementless THA. Such an unfavorable outcome can be related to several factors, including misdiagnosis of the original source, extrinsic causes, or post-revision/ETO THA pain. In this case, the patient had an extrinsic source of pain (chronic low back pain) and was on preoperative narcotic therapy, which likely reduced his pain tolerance. Evaluation of his lumbar spine before revision revealed degenerative disk disease and tenderness to palpation along the low back and sacroiliac joints. The patient's symptoms were unchanged after the revision, and passive range of motion of the hip was painless, suggesting that the low back was likely to be the source of his persistent symptoms. In such cases, it is important to counsel patients preoperatively that although their hip pain may be improved with revision surgery, symptoms related to the low back and lumbar spine will likely remain unchanged.

STRATEGIES TO MINIMIZE COMMON COMPLICATIONS

As demonstrated by the case presented here, evaluation of the patient with a painful THA is complicated

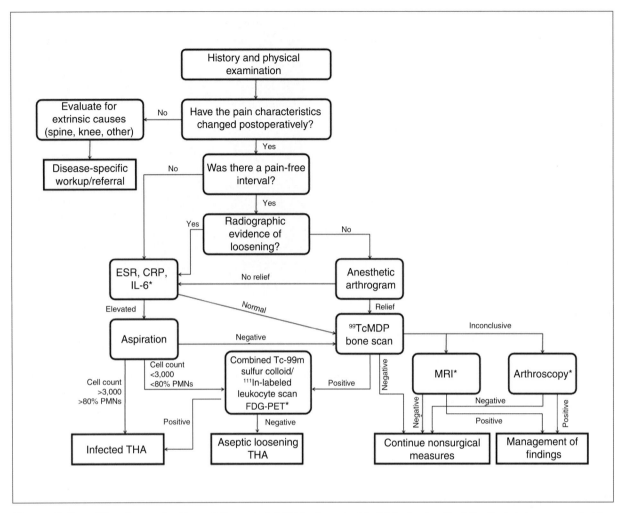

Figure 6 Algorithm for evaluation of the painful THA. An asterisk (*) indicates that limited data are available to support the use of this modality.

and challenging for both the surgeon and patient. Following an algorithm (**Figure 6**) allows an efficient and complete diagnostic workup, minimizing unnecessary tests and patient frustration. Although improvements in modern technology (MRI, arthroscopy, PET scans, and laboratory tests) make it possible to obtain more accurate diagnoses in a timely manner, several outpatient visits with serial physical examinations, blood draws, and radiographic studies may be required to identify the most likely source of pain.

When a clearly defined source of pain is identified, revision surgery to correct or treat the condition is warranted. On the other hand, surgical intervention is not indicated when a clear diagnosis is not found. Revision surgery carries substantial risks, and patients should be counseled regarding the diagnosis of the source of their pain and the treatment options available. Surgical intervention without a specific diagnosis can lead to continued pain and an unsatisfied patient. Nonsurgical measures are indicated in these patients until a definitive, treatable diagnosis is confirmed.

Routine postoperative surveillance of THA patients, including clinical and radiographic evaluation, should take place at regular intervals. Close follow-up allows early evaluation of osteolysis, aseptic loosening, polyethylene wear, and soft-tissue derangements. Appropriately timed interventions for these diagnoses may prevent patients from developing a painful THA. For example, patients with significant periprosthetic bone loss and a loose femoral component can be treated with an early revision to prevent future periprosthetic fracture. Similarly, progressive polyethylene wear (particularly in the setting of expansile osteolysis) recognized early may prevent subsequent pain from instability, osteolytic lesions, fractures through weakened bone, or particulate-induced synovitis. Periprosthetic joint infections should also be treated surgically in a timely manner to prevent sepsis and progressive bone loss.

The results of surgical treatment of thigh pain in the presence of a well-fixed femoral compo-

nent, iliopsoas tendinitis, trochanteric bursitis, or pain of unclear etiology are unpredictable at best, as is demonstrated by the case presented here. Patients with a preoperative history of chronic pain requiring long-term narcotic treatment, fibromyalgia, or anxiety may continue to experience pain after revision THA despite appropriate treatment for the intrinsic source of pain. It is important to follow a consistent algorithm during the diagnostic workup to avoid missing a potentially identifiable or treatable condition. If the etiology of the pain remains unclear after a thorough evaluation, referral to another orthopaedic surgeon or another physician (spine surgeon, vascular surgeon, neurologist, or general surgeon) for a second opinion may be helpful in coming to a definitive diagnosis.

REFERENCES

1. Britton AR, Murray DW, Bulstrode CJ, McPherson K, Denham RA: Pain levels after total hip replacement: Their use as endpoints for survival analysis. *J Bone Joint Surg Br* 1997;79: 93-98.

2. Kurtz S, Ong K, Lau E, Mowat F, Halpern M: Projections of primary and revision hip and knee arthroplasty in the United States from 2005 to 2030. *J Bone Joint Surg Am* 2007;89:780-785.

3. Bozic KJ, Rubash HE: The painful total hip replacement. *Clin Orthop Relat Res* 2004;420: 18-25.

4. Hamadouche M, Zniber B, Dumaine V, Kerboull M, Courpied JP: Reattachment of the ununited greater trochanter following total hip arthroplasty: The use of a trochanteric claw plate. *J Bone Joint Surg Am* 2003;85:1330-1337.

5. Bohl WR, Steffee AD: Lumbar spinal stenosis: A cause of continued pain and disability in patients after total hip arthroplasty. *Spine* 1979;4:168-173.

6. Heaton K, Dorr LD: Surgical release of iliopsoas tendon for groin pain after total hip arthroplasty. *J Arthroplasty* 2002;17: 779-781.

7. Di Cesare PE, Chang E, Preston CF, Liu CJ: Serum interleukin-6 as a marker of periprosthetic infection following total hip and knee arthroplasty. *J Bone Joint Surg Am* 2005;87:1921-1927.

8. Schinsky MF, Della Valle CJ, Sporer SM, Paprosky WG: Perioperative testing for joint infection in patients undergoing revision total hip arthroplasty. *J Bone Joint Surg Am* 2008; 90:1869-1875.

9. Spangehl MJ, Masri BA, O'Connell JX, Duncan CP: Prospective analysis of preoperative and intraoperative investigations for the diagnosis of infection at the sites of two hundred and two revision total hip arthroplasties. *J Bone Joint Surg Am* 1999; 81:672-683.

10. Bottner F, Wegner A, Winkelmann W, Becker K, Erren M, Gotze C: Interleukin-6, procalcitonin and

TNF-alpha: Markers of peri-prosthetic infection following total joint replacement. *J Bone Joint Surg Br* 2007;89:94-99.

11. Engh CA, Massin P, Suthers KE: Roentgenographic assessment of the biologic fixation of porous-surfaced femoral components. *Clin Orthop Relat Res* 1990; 257:107-128.

12. Harris WH, McGann WA: Loosening of the femoral component after use of the medullary-plug cementing technique: Follow-up note with a minimum five-year follow-up. *J Bone Joint Surg Am* 1986;68:1064-1066.

13. Udomkiat P, Wan Z, Dorr LD: Comparison of preoperative radiographs and intraoperative findings of fixation of hemispheric porous-coated sockets. *J Bone Joint Surg Am* 2001;83:1865-1870.

14. Yoder SA, Brand RA, Pedersen DR, O'Gorman TW: Total hip acetabular component position affects component loosening rates. *Clin Orthop Relat Res* 1988;228: 79-87.

15. Hodgkinson JP, Shelley P, Wroblewski BM: The correlation between the roentgenographic appearance and operative findings at the bone-cement junction of the socket in Charnley low friction arthroplasties. *Clin Orthop Relat Res* 1988;228:105-109.

16. Hartofilakidis G, Georgiades G, Babis GC: A comparison of the outcome of cemented all-polyethylene and cementless metal-backed acetabular sockets in primary total hip arthroplasty. *J Arthroplasty* 2008: March 27 [epub ahead of print].

17. DeLee JG, Charnley J: Radiological demarcation of cemented sockets in total hip replacement. *Clin Orthop Relat Res* 1976;121:20-32.

18. Ali F, Wilkinson JM, Cooper JR, et al: Accuracy of joint aspiration for the preoperative diagnosis of infection in total hip arthroplasty. *J Arthroplasty* 2006;21:221-226.

19. Williams JL, Norman P, Stockley I: The value of hip aspiration versus tissue biopsy in diagnosing infection before exchange hip arthroplasty surgery. *J Arthroplasty* 2004;19:582-586.

20. Della Valle CJ, Zuckerman JD, Di Cesare PE: Periprosthetic sepsis. *Clin Orthop Relat Res* 2004; 420:26-31.

21. Ghanem E, Parvizi J, Burnett RS, et al: Cell count and differential of aspirated fluid in the diagnosis of infection at the site of total knee arthroplasty. *J Bone Joint Surg Am* 2008;90:1637-1643.

22. Salvati EA, Gonzalez Della Valle A, Masri BA, Duncan CP: The infected total hip arthroplasty. *Instr Course Lect* 2003;52:223-245.

23. Braunstein EM, Cardinal E, Buckwalter KA, Capello W: Bupivicaine arthrography of the post-arthroplasty hip. *Skeletal Radiol* 1995;24:519-521.

24. McCarthy JC, Jibodh SR, Lee JA: The role of arthroscopy in evaluation of painful hip arthroplasty. *Clin Orthop Relat Res* 2008: October 8, [epub ahead of print].

25. Mittal R, Khetarpal R, Malhotra R, Kumar R: The role of Tc-99m bone imaging in the management of pain after complicated total hip replacement. *Clin Nucl Med* 1997;22:593-595.

26. Oswald SG, Van Nostrand D, Savory CG, Callaghan JJ: Three-phase bone scan and indium white blood cell scintigraphy following porous coated hip arthroplasty: A prospective study of the prosthetic tip. *J Nucl Med* 1989;30: 1321-1331.

27. Lieberman JR, Huo MH, Schneider R, Salvati EA, Rodi S: Evaluation of painful hip arthroplasties: Are technetium bone scans necessary? *J Bone Joint Surg Br* 1993;75:475-478.

28. Nagoya S, Kaya M, Sasaki M, Tateda K, Yamashita T: Diagnosis of peri-prosthetic infection at the hip using triple-phase bone scintigraphy. *J Bone Joint Surg Br* 2008;90:140-144.

29. Merkel KD, Brown ML, Dewanjee MK, Fitzgerald RH Jr: Comparison of indium-labeled-leukocyte imaging with sequential technetium-gallium scanning in the diagnosis of low-grade musculoskeletal sepsis: A prospective study. *J Bone Joint Surg Am* 1985;67:465-476.

30. Scher DM, Pak K, Lonner JH, Finkel JE, Zuckerman JD, Di Cesare PE: The predictive value of indium-111 leukocyte scans in the diagnosis of infected total hip, knee, or resection arthroplasties. *J Arthroplasty* 2000;15:295-300.

31. Pill SG, Parvizi J, Tang PH, et al: Comparison of fluorodeoxyglucose positron emission tomography and (111) indium-white blood cell imaging in the diagnosis of periprosthetic infection of the hip. *J Arthroplasty* 2006;21(6, Suppl 2)91-97.

32. Cooper HJ, Ranawat AS, Potter HG, Foo LF, Jawetz ST, Ranawat CS: Magnetic resonance imaging in the diagnosis and management of hip pain after total hip arthroplasty. *J Arthroplasty* 2008; August 8 [epub ahead of print].

33. Potter HG, Nestor BJ, Sofka CM, Ho ST, Peters LE, Salvati EA: Magnetic resonance imaging after total hip arthroplasty: Evaluation of periprosthetic soft tissue. *J Bone Joint Surg Am* 2004;86: 1947-1954.

34. Weiland DE, Walde TA, Leung SB, et al: Magnetic resonance imaging in the evaluation of periprosthetic acetabular osteolysis: A cadaveric study. *J Orthop Res* 2005;23: 713-719.

INDEX

Page numbers followed by *f* indicate figures; page numbers followed by *t* indicate tables.